How to Play Basketball For Kids

A Guide for Parents and Players

Author Tony R. Smith

Copyright © 2019 by Tony R. Smith. All Rights Reserved. No part of this publication may be reproduced, distributed, or transmitted in any form or by any means, including photocopying, recording, or other electronic or mechanical methods, or by any information storage and retrieval system without the prior written permission of S.S. Publishing, except in the case of very brief quotations embodied in critical reviews and certain other noncommercial uses permitted by copyright law

Table of Contents

Introduction 7
   Practice Dribbling. 8
   Practice Passing and Catching 9
   Practice Footwork 10
Health Benefits of Playing Basketball 11
   Promotes Cardiovascular Health 12
   Burns Calories 12
   Builds Bone Strength. 13
   Boosts the Immune System 14
   Provides Strength Training 14
   Boosts Mental Development 15
   Develops Better Coordination and Motor Skills
   16
   Develops Self-Discipline and Concentration ... 17
   Improves Awareness of Space and Body 17
   Boosts Confidence 18
History of Basketball 20

- The 12 Rules of Basketball 23
- The First Game of Basketball Ever Played 26
- Rules of Basketball 29
  - Fouls 33
  - Violations 36
  - Player Positions 39
- Basic Skills of Basketball 41
  - Dribbling. 42
  - Passing 43
  - Shooting 44
  - Rebounding 46
  - Defense 47
- Drills. 48
  - Shooting Drills. 48
    - 21 Cones – Shooting Drill 49
    - Pivot Shooting – Shooting Drill 51
    - Chase Down Layups – Shooting Drill 52
    - Pressure – Shooting Drill 53
  - Dribbling Drills. 54
    - Dribbling Lines – Dribbling Drill 54
    - Dribble Knockout – Dribbling Drill 56
    - Collision Dribbling – Dribbling Drill 57
    - Scarecrow Tiggy – Dribbling Drill 58

Dribble Tag – Dribbling Drill 59
Sharks and Minnows – Dribbling Drill 60
Passing Drills 61
  Partner Passing – Passing Drill 61
  Stationary Keepings Off – Passing Drill 61
  Count Em' Up – Passing Drill 62
  Continuous 3 on 2 – Passing Drill 64
Footwork Drills 66
  Four Corners – Footwork Drill 67
  Red Light, Green Light – Footwork Drill 66
  Explode, Pivot, Pass – Footwork Drill 68
Partner Drills 70
  Close Out Drill 70
  Box Out Drill 71
  One on One Drill 72
  Elbow Shooting 73
Strength and Conditioning Drills 74
  Plyo Push Ups 74
  Medicine Ball Throws 75
    Medicine Ball Rotation Throws 75
    Medicine Ball Slams 75
    Medicine Ball Squat Throws 76
  Cool Down Drills 76

- Walking Without Shoes 77
- Practice Good Form 77
- Single Knee Cross 77
- Ankle Rotations 78
- Shoulder and Neck 78
- Calves ....,............................. 79

Defensive Drills 80
- Defensive Mirrors – Defense Drill 80
- Defensive Specialist – Defense Drill 83
- One-on-One – Defense Drill 85
- Zig-Zag Slides – Defensive Drill 86

Fun Drills 87
- War – Fun Drill 87
- Golden Child – Fun Drill 88
- Elimination – Fun Drill 90
- Small-Sided Games – Fun Drill 91
- Game-Winner – Fun Game 92

Drills Every Basketball Player Should Master ... 93
- Full Speed Shooting. 95
- Cutt off(1 on 1 Closeouts) 96
- Defensive Lane Slides 97
- Two Ball Passing 98
- Curl, Fade, Cut 99

- Two-Ball Dribbling 101
- Mikan/Reverse Mikan 103
- Post "Crab" Dribble Moves. 106
- Full Speed Dribbling 108
- Muscle Memory Shooting 110
- Eating Right 111
  - Carbohydrates 113
  - Protein 116
  - Fat 118
  - Pregame Meals 119
  - Fueling During Games 120
  - Recovery 123
- Agility Drills (Improve Jumping Ability) 127
  - Jump rope 126
  - Box Jumps 131
- Conclusion 135
- Basketball Stats Tracker 138
- Disclaimer Statement 148

Introduction

The game of basketball is an exciting sport- it is fun, great for exercise, and children learn important lessons that can be applied to other aspects of life. The good news for parents eager to get their children involved in this athletic activity is that basketball can be introduced at a very young age. Basic motor and co-ordination skills such as dribbling (bouncing) a ball and shooting can be introduced when a child is just a couple years old.

Youth leagues accept children starting around age five or six: an excellent time for children to begin learning the fundamentals of the game. Concepts such as hustle, teamwork, sportsmanship, and attitude can be introduced, as can more technical aspects of the game; such as footwork, defense, and shooting mechanics.

Practice Dribbling

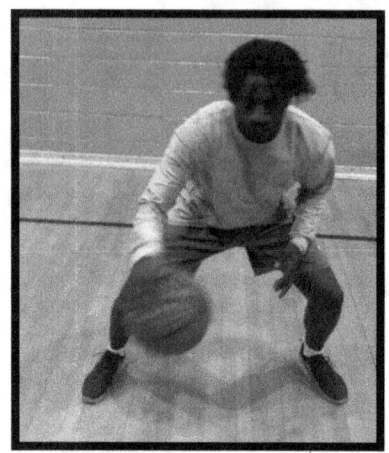 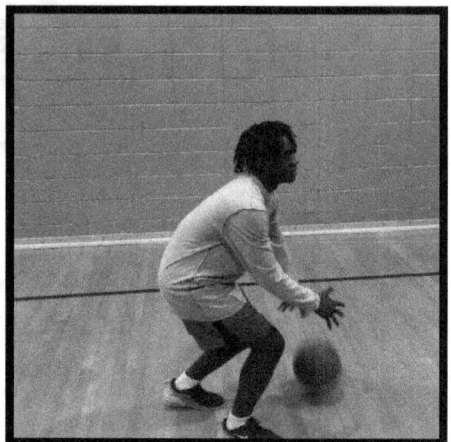

Young players must develop confidence and a feel for the ball. It is important for a player to be able to dribble with either hand and to maintain a dribble despite obstacles. Speed while dribbling is important and young players can have races and even play tag, while they are dribbling a ball, to improve their overall dribbling ability.

Using a mini ball, younger players can develop dribbling through practice techniques such as hip circles, leg circles, ankle circles, and neck circles. They should consistently practice all aspects of dribbling: right-handed and left-handed dribbling, dribbling with their heads up, switching hands while dribbling, dribbling around cones and chairs your in the driveway.

Practice Passing and Catching

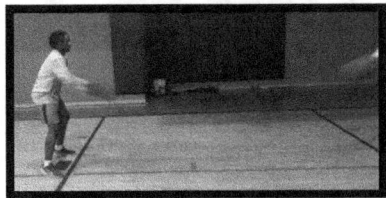 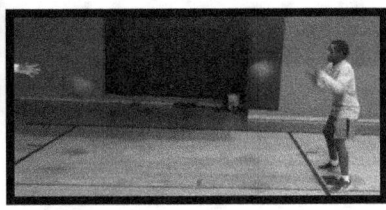

Young players must learn how to pass and catch the ball properly. They should practice a variety of passes: two-hand passes from the chest, one-hand baseball passes, two-hand bounce passes, and over-the-head passes. At the same time, it is suggested players work on catching the ball with two hands. [Technique tip: players should be taught to catch the ball in an athletic position; with their knees bent; their hands making a target-chest level high; and their feet balanced, shoulder width apart.

Practice Footwork

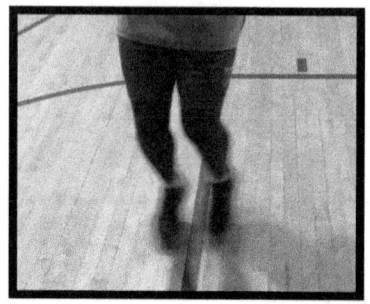 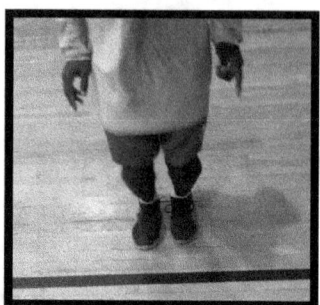

Basic footwork is the foundation of good play and an appropriate area of focus for young players. Developing players may not be ready to make a ball fake or jab step and dribble drive to the basket, but they can practice the footwork for these moves and learn to execute them.

Basically, children can begin to play as soon as they express an interest in the game. While young players learn the fundamentals, they develop a passion for the game that could last a lifetime.

Health Benefits of Playing Basketball

Basketball is a much-loved sport across the world because it can be played as a competitive sport or a casual game on the local court. It is also a great way to work out as it involves using your entire body. If you want a sport that helps you stay fit and healthy, basketball is the perfect choice as it comes with several health benefits.

Promotes Cardiovascular Health

Basketball is great for your heart health! It is a fast-paced game that involves a good deal of jumping and running; which is a fantastic way to keep moving and increase your heart rate. It also helps in building endurance to ensure your heart is healthy. This has been shown to lower the risk of stroke and heart disease later in life.

Burns Calories

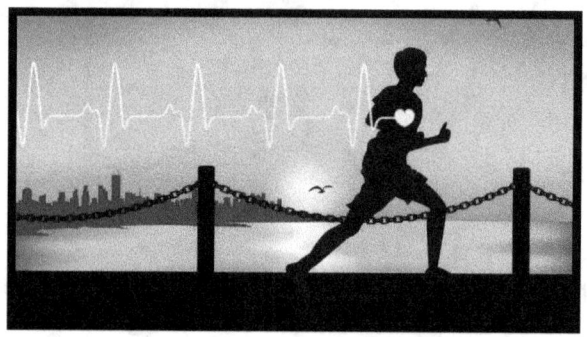

Do you want to shed a few extra kilos? Play basketball! All the quick lateral movements- running and jumping- give you an aerobic workout that in turn can help you burn a great deal of calories. For every hour of basketball, a person who weighs 165 pounds can expect to burn about 600 calories while a person who weighs 250 pounds can expect to burn approximately 900 calories.

Builds Bone Strength

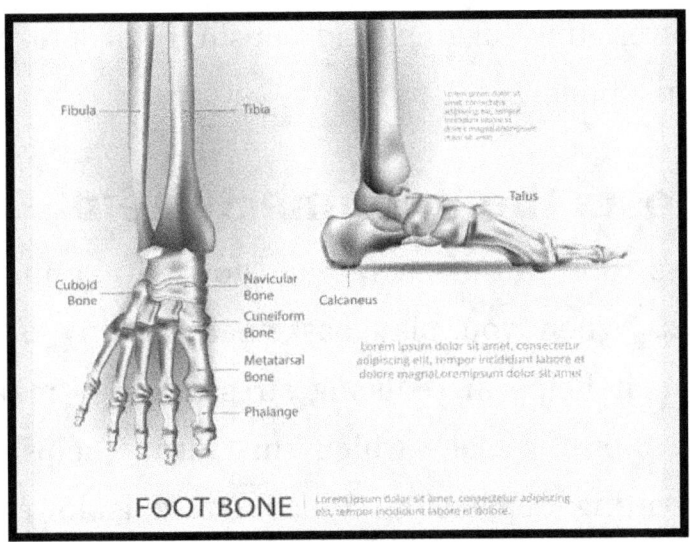

The physical demands of this awesome sport help in improving and building bone strength. Any physical activity that involves weight-bearing allows the formation of new bone tissue, and this, in turn, makes the bones stronger.

Muscles and bones in your body become stronger with basketball as it is a physical activity that involves the tugging and pushing of muscles against bone.

Boosts the Immune System

Stress robs you of energy and focus to complete tasks. When you play basketball or any other sport, it helps in reducing stress. It also makes you more social, which in turns helps in preventing depression. When stress is lowered, your immune system gets a boost as well.

Provides Strength Training

The development of lean muscle can be supported by playing basketball. You get an excellent full-body workout that can develop your lower back, neck, deltoids, traps and core muscles. Basketball also makes your legs stronger, and the movements like shooting and dribbling help strengthen your arms, hand muscles and wrist flexors.

Boosts Mental Development

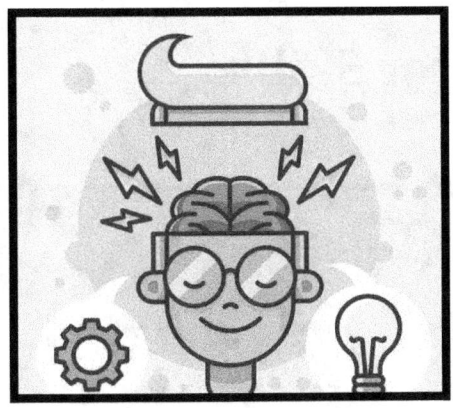

Basketball may be a fast-paced game that utilizes an abundance of physical skills, but it is also a brain game that requires you to "think on your toes." It requires you to have focus so that you can accurately and quickly process the action on the court and make decisions that are effective with the ball. It also requires you to train yourself so that you can observe your opponents and teammates constantly and make quick decisions based on their actions.

Develops Better Coordination and Motor Skills

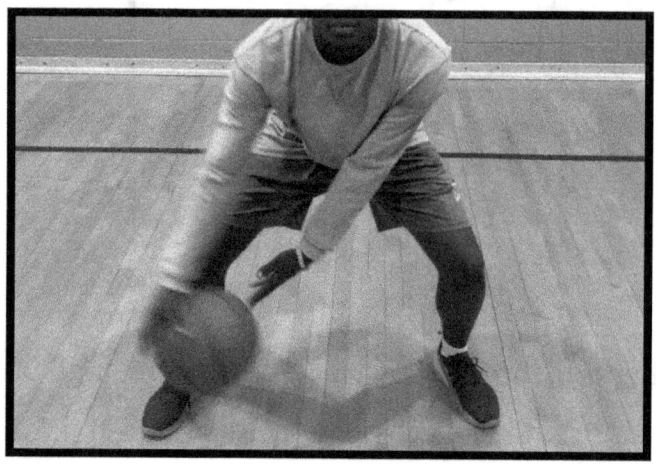

Basketball training helps develop excellent hand-eye coordination as well as full-body coordination. Dribbling practice provides training for hand-eye coordination; while practicing rebounding missed shots develops full-body coordination.

Develops Self-Discipline and Concentration

As with other sports, there are rules to follow while playing basketball. Breaking these rules, can lead to personal and/or team penalties. Sticking to structure, helps you develop self- discipline, which is important; as it supports competition and fairness, at the same time. It also keeps your mind focused and alert.

Improves Awareness of Space and Body

You need to know where you are positioned to make that perfect shot or play defense effectively. When you have an awareness of the space and body, you will know exactly where you need to be when your teammate or opponent makes a shot or passes the ball. When your spatial awareness is improved, it also helps in keeping you in balance.

Boosts Confidence

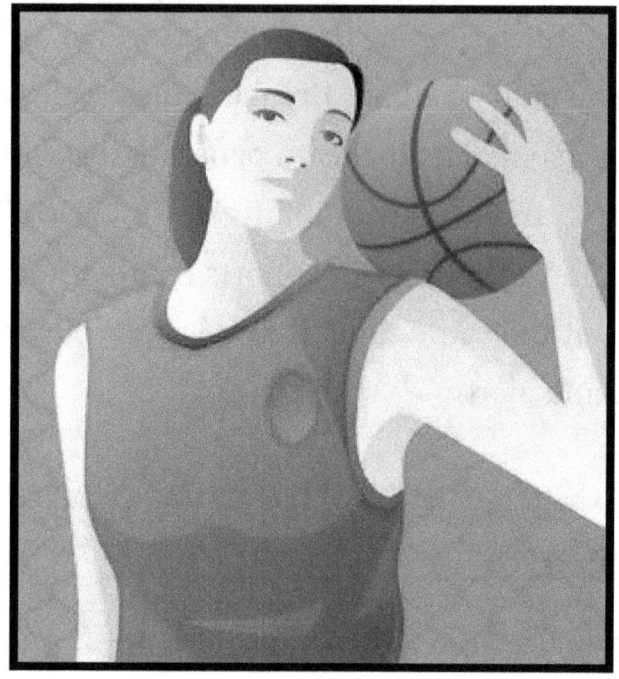

Being a good player and team member increases your self- esteem and confidence. When confidence is boosted, your faith in your skills is also increased. The overall effect of being more confident allows you to face life with an improved disposition and this increase has a positive effect on every aspect of your life.

The fast-paced action involved in basketball makes it one of the most exciting games to play and watch in the world. The fact that it provides numerous total health benefits is an excellent bonus. It is no wonder that the 44th President of the US has made it a part of his regular workout regimen to keep himself physically and mentally fit. It is a great game for both adults and children. If you are looking to play a sport that gives you multiple benefits, inside and out, this is the one for you.

Basketball can be played alone or with friends – no matter what you choose, you get a great workout and ensure that you stay physically and mentally fit and active for many years. With the many fitness benefits of basketball, it is the perfect reason for to pick up a ball and start shooting some hoops.

History of Basketball

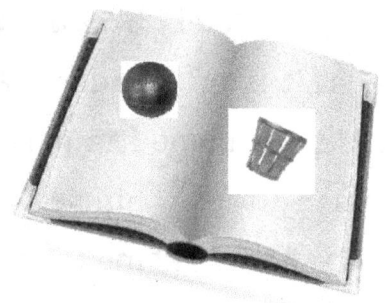

The game of basketball originated in December 1891 by James Naismith. Canadian born, Naismith was a teacher at the YMCA training school in Springfield, Massachusetts. He was required to train young men to become instructors at newly opened YMCA centers.

With the cold weather keeping the class indoors, in December 1891, Naismith was asked by the schools Superintendent of Physical Education, Dr. Luther. H. Gulick, to create an indoor game that would keep the young men active during the cold winter months.

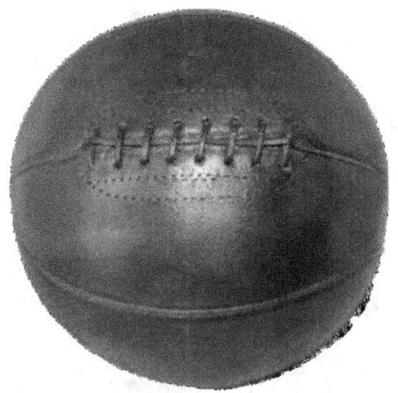

Upon this request, Naismith nervously set out to create a game that his class would enjoy. In a diary found many years later he had written:

"I felt this was a crucial moment in my life as it meant success or failure of my attempt to hold the interest of the class and devise a new game"

With the help of his wife and memories of playing 'Duck on a Rock' during his childhood, he decided to create a game that would focus on skill rather than strength.

For those who are curious, 'Duck on a Rock' was a game in which players threw rocks at a certain target placed on top of a large boulder or tree stump.

The game he ended up inventing is the game we all know and love today – basketball.

Basketball required very little equipment to play... two peach baskets hanging 10 feet above the ground, and a soccer ball.

The object of the game was to work as a team to throw or bat the soccer ball into the opposing teams peach basket, while defending a score in your peach basket from the opposition.

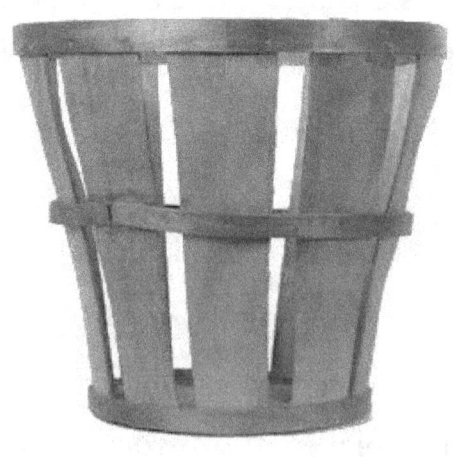

As you can imagine, it was a major pain getting the ball out of the peach basket when a team finally scored. Some say they used a long pole to push the ball out, others say someone was required to climb a ladder to retrieve it.

Either way, the initial players weren't great shooters so they didn't have to worry about this too much. Heck, in the first game ever played, there was only one score during the entire game!

Originally the game involved nine players on each team. You might wonder why nine?! This is because Naismith's class had 18 people in it.

He also developed rules for the game known as 'The 12 Rules of Basketball'.

The 12 Rules of Basketball

- ✓ The ball may be thrown in any direction with one or both hands.
- ✓ The ball may be batted in any direction with one or both hands, but never with the fist.

- A player cannot run with the ball. The player must throw it from the spot on which he catches it, allowance to be made for a man running at good speed.
- The ball must be held by the hands. The arms or body must not be used for holding it.
- No shouldering, holding, pushing, striking or tripping in any way of an opponent. The first infringement of this rule by any person shall count as a foul; the second shall disqualify him until the next goal is made or, if there was evident intent to injure the person, for the whole of the game. No substitution shall be allowed.
- A foul is striking at the ball with the fist, violations of Rules 3 and 4 and such as described in Rule 5.
- If either side makes three consecutive fouls it shall count as a goal for the opponents (consecutive means without the opponents in the meantime making a foul).

- ✓ A goal shall be made when the ball is thrown or batted from the grounds into the basket and stays there, providing those defending the goal do no touch or disturb the goal. If the ball rests on the edges, and the opponent moves the basket, it shall count as a goal.
- ✓ When the ball goes out of bounds, it shall be thrown into the field and played by the first person touching it. In case of dispute, the umpire shall throw it straight into the field. The thrower-in is allowed five seconds. If he holds it longer, it shall go to the opponent. If any side persists in delaying the game, the umpire shall call a foul on them.
- ✓ The umpire shall be the judge of the men and shall note the fouls and notify the referee when three consecutive fouls have been made. He shall have power to disqualify men according to Rule 5.
- ✓ The referee shall be judge of the ball and shall decide when the ball is in play, in

bounds, to which side it belongs, and shall keep the time. He shall decide when a goal has been made and keep account of the goals, with any other duties that are usually performed by a referee.

- ✓ The time shall be two fifteen-minute halves, with five minutes rest between.

The First Game of Basketball Ever Played

The first game of basketball was played on the 21st of December, 1891, at the YMCA training school in Springfield, Massachusetts.

The gym was incredibly small. Only 50 feet x 35 feet, compared to current day courts which are 94 feet x 53 feet.

Naismith arrived early that day. Little did he know he was about to create basketball history.

After posting the '13 Rules of Basketball' on the bulletin board of the gym, he then nailed a peach basket to the lower rail of the balcony on both ends of the gym.

When the players arrived, Naismith split his eighteen students into two teams of nine players. He had done his best to teach them the 13 rules of basketball. They were now ready to embark on a game destined to change sports forever.

Little did James Naismith or of any of his players realize how big this new game would become in a very short amount of time. The players involved in the first basketball game were;

Team 1:

John J. Thompson; Eugene S. Libby; T. Duncan Patton; Frank Mahan; Finlay G. MacDonald; William H. Davis; Lyman Archibald; Edwin P. Ruggles; and William R. Chase.

Team 2:

George Weller; Wilbert Carey; Ernest Hildner; Raymond Kaighn; Genzabaro Ishikawa; Benjamin S. French; Franklin Barnes; George Day and Henry Gelan.

The final score of the game ended ,1 – 0 with Team 1 as the victors.

William R. Chase scored the only goal of the game from 25 feet away from the basket, becoming the first person to score a goal during a game in basketball history!

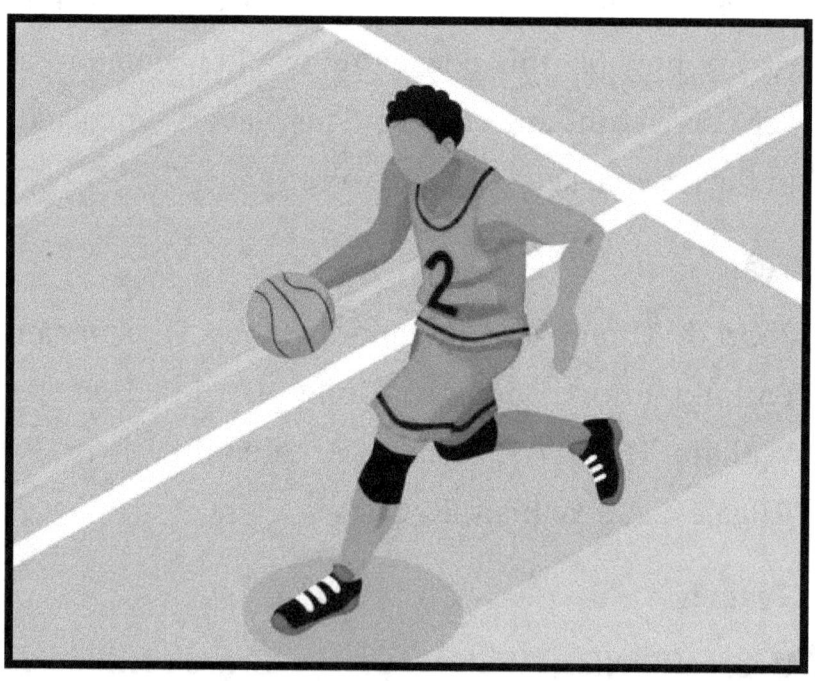

Rules of Basketball

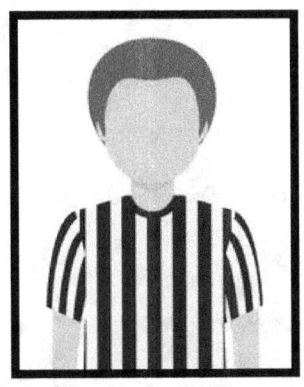

The rules of basketball, thankfully, are fairly straightforward. However, for the younger players, some rules can be easily forgotten. The three-second rule addressing how long an offensive player can be in the key before clearing out is a good example.

Basketball is a team sport. Two teams of five players each try to score by shooting a ball through a hoop elevated 10 feet above the ground. The game is played on a rectangular floor called the court, and there is a hoop at each end. The court is divided into two main sections by the mid-court line. If the offensive team puts the ball into play behind the mid-court line, it has ten seconds to get the ball over the mid-court line. If it doesn't, then the defense gets the ball. Once the offensive team gets the ball over the mid-court line, it can no longer have possession of the ball in the area in back of the line. If it does, the defense is awarded the ball.

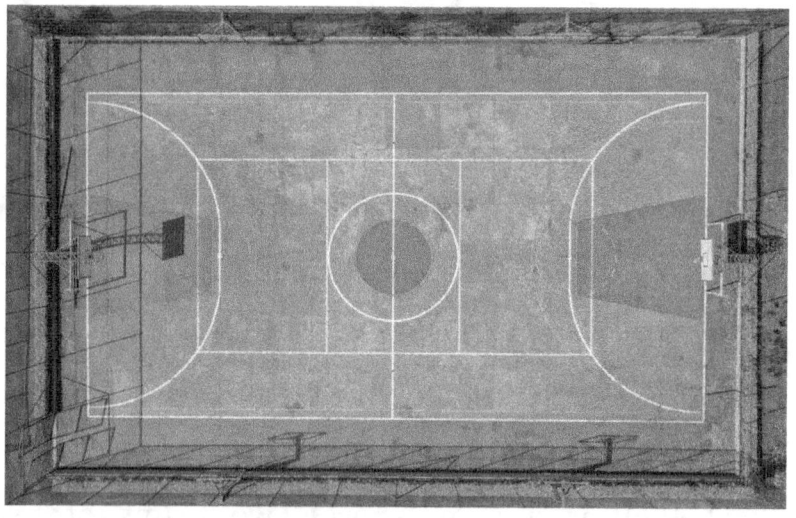

The ball is moved down the court toward the basket by passing or dribbling. The team with the ball is called the offense. The team without the ball is called the defense. They try to steal the ball, contest shots, steal and deflect passes, and garner rebounds.

When a team makes a basket, they score two points and the ball goes to the other team. If a basket, or field goal, is made outside of the three-point arc, then that basket is worth three points. A free throw is worth one point. Free throws are awarded to a team according to some formats involving the number of fouls committed in a half and/or the type of foul committed. Fouling a shooter always results in two or three free throws being awarded the shooter, depending upon where he was when he shot the ball. If he was beyond the three-point line, then he gets three shots. Other types of fouls do not result in free throws being awarded until a certain number have accumulated during a half. Once that number is reached, then the player who was fouled is awarded a '1-and-1' opportunity. If he makes his first free throw, he gets to attempt a second. If he misses the first shot, the ball is live on the rebound.

Each game is divided into sections. All levels have two halves. In college, each half is twenty minutes long. In high school and below, the halves are divided into eight (and sometimes, six) minute quarters. In the pros, quarters are twelve minutes long. There is a gap of several minutes between halves. Gaps between quarters are relatively short. If the score is tied at the end of regulation, then overtime periods of various lengths are played until a winner emerges.

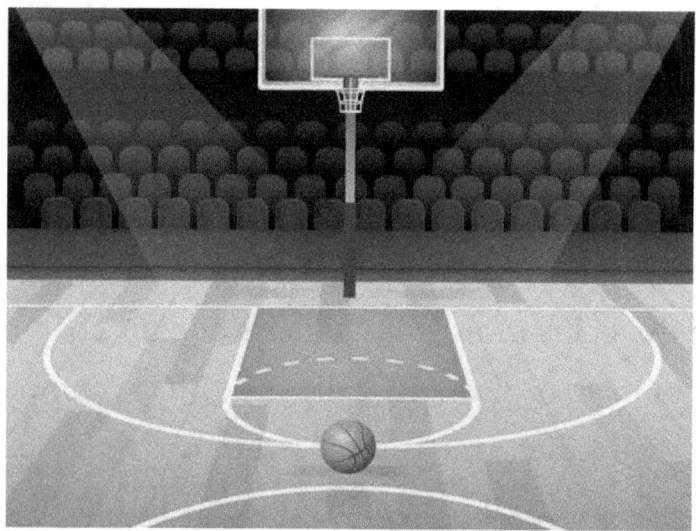

Each team is assigned a basket or goal to defend. This means that the other basket is their scoring basket. At halftime, the teams switch goals. The game begins with one player from either team at center court. A referee will toss the ball up between the two. The player that gets his hands on the ball will tip it to a teammate. This is called a tip-off. In addition to stealing the ball from an opposing player, there are other ways for a team to get the ball. One such way is if the other team commits a foul or violation.

Fouls

Personal fouls: Personal fouls include any type of illegal physical contact.

- ✓ Hitting
- ✓ Pushing
- ✓ Slapping
- ✓ Holding
- ✓ Illegal pick/screen – [when an offensive player is moving] When an offensive player sticks out a limb and makes physical contact with a defender in an attempt to block the path of the defender.

Personal foul penalties: If a player is shooting while being fouled, then he gets two free throws if his shot doesn't go in, but only one free throw if his shot does go in.

- ✓ Three free throws are awarded if the player is fouled while shooting for a three-point goal and they miss their shot. If a player is fouled while shooting a three-point shot and makes it anyway, he is awarded one free throw. Thus, he could score four points on the play.
- ✓ Inbounds. If fouled while not shooting, the ball is given to the team the foul was committed upon. They get the ball at the nearest side or baseline, out of bounds, and have 5 seconds to pass the ball onto the court.
- ✓ One & one. If the team committing the foul has seven or more fouls in the game, then the player who was fouled is awarded one free throw. If he makes his first shot, then he is awarded another free throw.

- ✓ Ten or more fouls. If the team committing the foul has ten or more fouls, then the fouled player receives two free throws.

Charging. An offensive foul that is committed when a player pushes or runs over a defensive player. The ball is given to the team that the foul was committed upon.

Blocking. Blocking is illegal personal contact resulting from a defender not establishing position in time to prevent an opponent's drive to the basket.

Flagrant foul. Violent contact with an opponent. This includes hitting, kicking, and punching. This type of foul results in free throws plus the offense retaining possession of the ball after the free throws.

Intentional foul. When a player makes physical contact with another player with no reasonable effort to steal the ball. It is a judgment call for the officials.

Technical foul. Technical foul. A player or a coach can commit this type of foul. It does not involve player contact or the ball, but is instead about the 'manners' of the game. Foul language, obscenity, obscene gestures, and even arguing can be considered a technical foul, as can technical details regarding filling in the scorebook improperly or dunking during warm-ups.

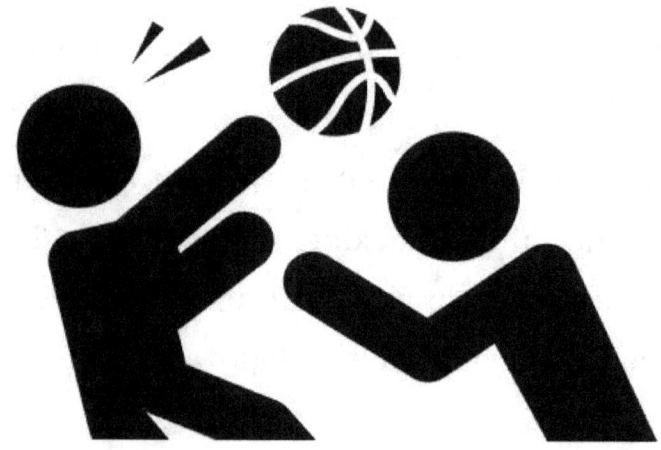

Violations

Walking/Traveling. Taking more than 'a step and a half' without dribbling the ball is traveling. Moving your pivot foot once you've stopped dribbling is traveling.

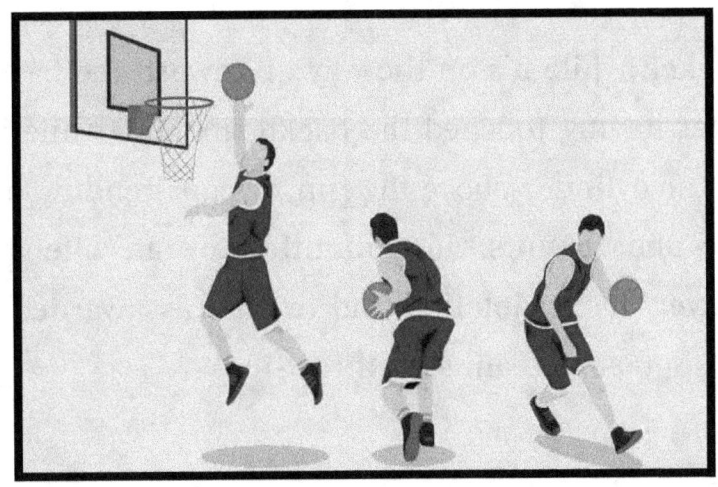

Carrying/palming. When a player dribbles the ball with his hand too far to the side of or, sometimes, even under the ball.

Double Dribble. Dribbling the ball with both hands on the ball at the same time or picking up the dribble and then dribbling again is a double dribble.

Held ball. Occasionally, two or more opposing players will gain possession of the ball at the same time. In order to avoid a prolonged and/or violent tussle, the referee stops the action and awards the ball to one team or the other on a rotating basis.

Goaltending. If a defensive player interferes with a shot while it's on the way down toward the basket, while it's on the way up toward the basket after having touched the backboard, or while it's in the cylinder above the rim, it's goaltending and the shot counts. If committed by an offensive player, it's a violation and the ball is awarded to the opposing team for a throw-in.

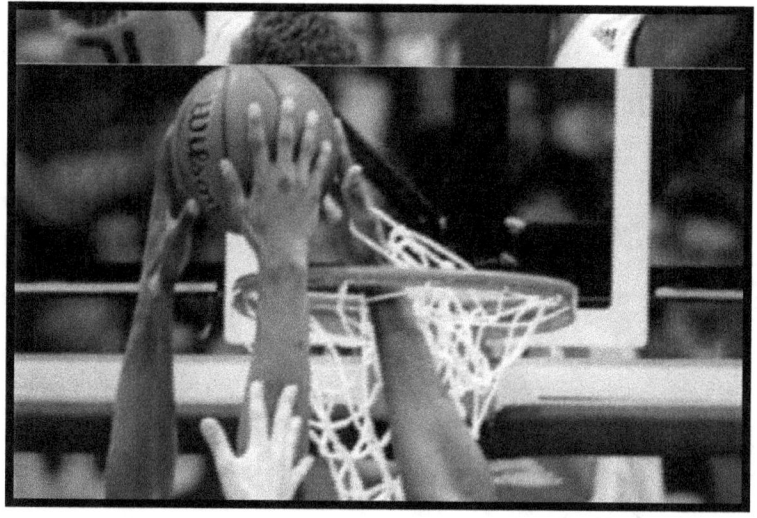

Backcourt violation. Once the offense has brought the ball across the mid-court line, they cannot go back across the line during possession. If they do, the ball is awarded to the other team to pass inbounds.

Time restrictions. A player passing the ball inbounds has five seconds to pass the ball. If he does not, then the ball is awarded to the other team. Other time restrictions include the rule that a player cannot have the ball for more than five seconds when being closely guarded and, in some states and levels, shot-clock restrictions requiring a team to attempt a shot within a given time frame.

Player Positions

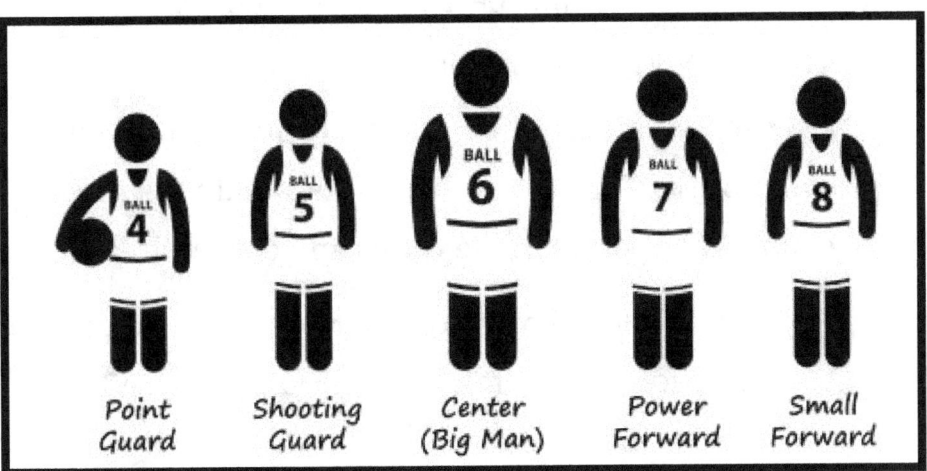

Center. Centers are generally your tallest players. They generally are positioned near the basket.

- ✓ Offensive – The center's goal is to get open for a pass and to shoot. They are also responsible for blocking defenders, known as picking or screening, to open other players up for driving to the basket for a goal. Centers are expected to get some offensive rebounds and put-backs.
- ✓ Defensive – On defense, the center's main responsibility is to keep opponents from shooting by blocking shots and passes in the key area. They also are expected to get a lot of rebounds because they're taller.

Forward. Your next tallest players will most likely be your forwards. While a forward may be called upon to play under the hoop, they may also be required to operate in the wings and corner areas.

- ✓ Offensive – Forwards are responsible to get free for a pass, take outside shots, drive for goals, and rebound.
- ✓ Defensive – Responsibilities include preventing drives to the goal and rebounding.

Guard. These are potentially your shortest players and they should be really good at dribbling fast, seeing the court, and passing. It is their job to bring the ball down the court and set up offensive plays.

- ✓ Offensive – Dribbling, passing, and setting up offensive plays are a guard's main responsibilities. They also need to be able to drive to the basket and to shoot from the perimeter.
- ✓ Defensive – On defense, a guard is responsible for stealing passes, contesting shots, preventing drives to the hoop, and for boxing out.

Basic Skills of Basketball

It is the rare basketball player who can do it all at the highest level. Michael Jordan, Magic Johnson and LeBron James were able to handle the ball, pass it, shoot it, rebound and play defense with the best of the best. If you excel at one or two of the five top basketball skills, there will be a place for you on most basketball courts. And if you excel at all five, the sky is the limit.

Basketball is a fast-paced game that requires the knowledge and instinct to perform quickly and properly. The sport of basketball requires five basic skills. While some players might be more experienced with some skills than others, it is best to have at least some ability in all five areas.

Dribbling

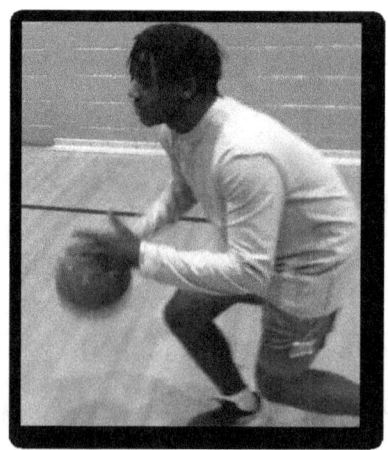 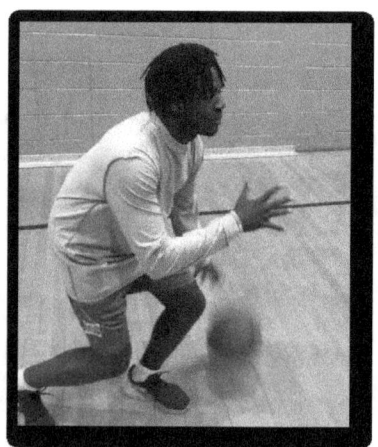

Good technique is critical for a ball handler. Top point guards dribble and control the ball as if it were on a string. Dribble with your fingertips rather than your palm and with your head up so you can see the opposition and your teammates. Keep your body low and use your off-ball hand to help keep your defender at bay. Work on dribbling with both hands, so you'll be comfortable going to your left as well as your right.

Passing

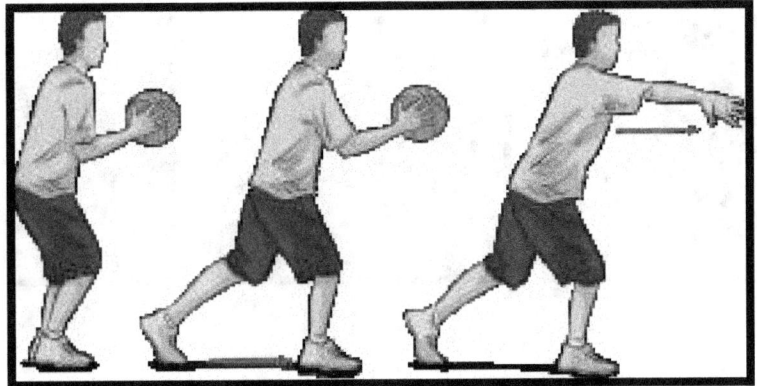

Great passers can see the whole court and anticipate where a teammate will go and what a defender will do. Mastering the basics is the place to start. Develop a two-hand chest pass, bounce pass, and overhead pass so you can deliver the ball to your teammates in the best position for them to shoot or beat their defender. Steve Nash or Derrick Rose can dazzle you with a behind-the-back or a no-look pass, but those moves are not just for show; they provide a teammate the best chance to score.

Shooting

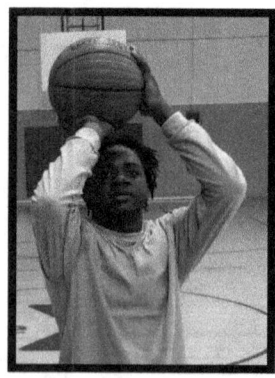
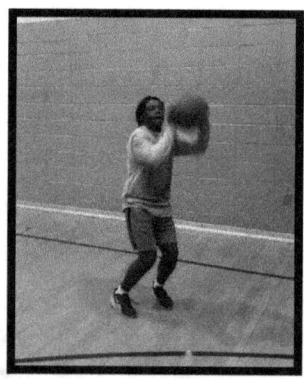
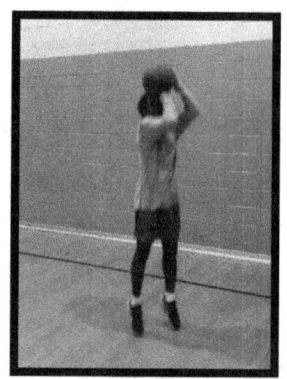

It's difficult to score if you can't shoot the ball effectively. As *Better Basketball Coaching*

explains, shooting is something of an art form, and some players, such as Kevin Durant and Ray Allen, have a knack for it; however, everyone can improve their shooting through proper technique and lots of practice. Proper technique includes squaring your body up to the target; shooting the ball with your fingertips; keeping your elbows from flying; putting backspin and arc on the shot and following through completely after letting the ball fly.

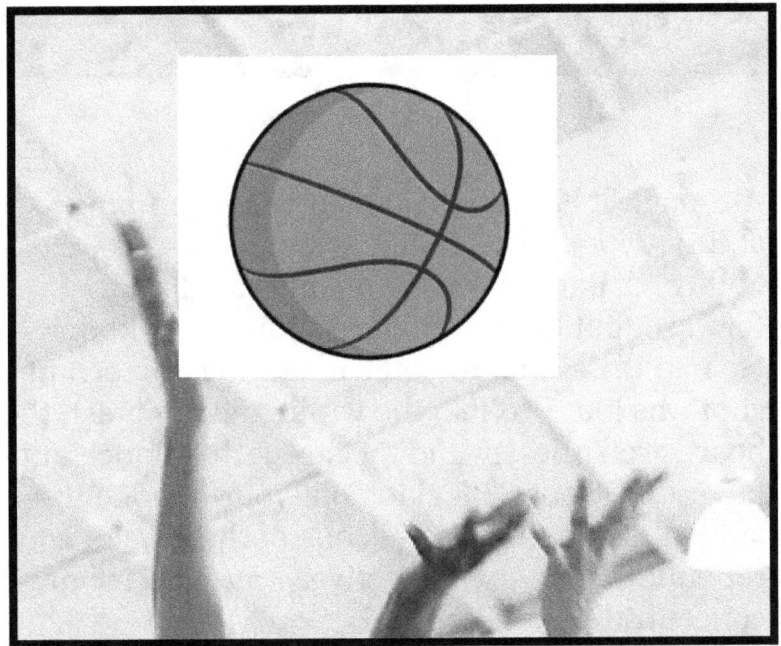

Rebounding

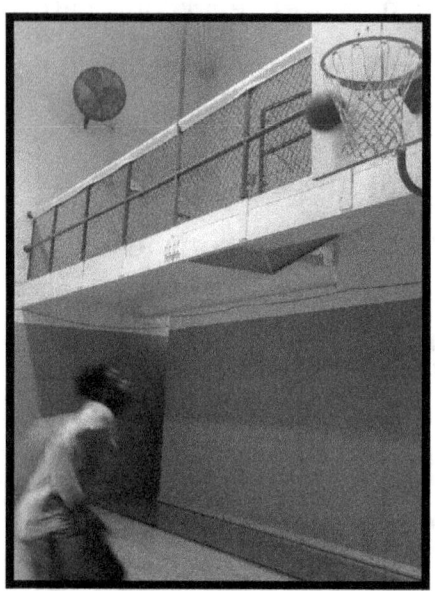 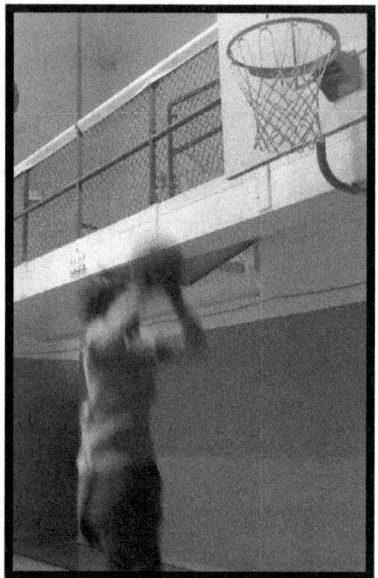

Although it helps to be tall and have jumping ability, rebounding is a matter of desire as well as ability. C. Barkley was relatively small for a forward, but he was an outstanding rebounder. He had the ability to determine where an errant shot was likely to fall, the willingness to crash the boards relentlessly and the strength to block out taller opponents. Blocking out your opponent -- also called boxing out -- is one of the keys to good rebounding. To do it effectively, maintain your concentration and focus.

Defense

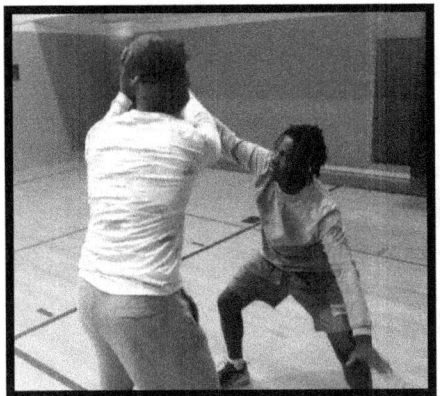 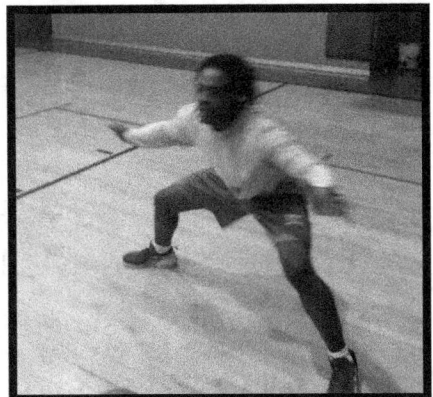

Even the best scorers go into shooting slumps, but you can always play good defense if you hustle and understand both individual and team defense. When you are defending a player, keep you head lower than his. Stay close enough to the offensive player to bother him -- but not so close he can blow by you with one step. Know your opponent's tendencies so you can dictate the direction you want him to move. Be aware of the other players on the court, so you can play "help defense" when a teammate loses his man.

Drills

Shooting Drills

This is a great drill for players to practice shooting with perfect form and also a drill for coaches to teach and correct shooting form.

Players form three lines a couple of feet out from the basket. Use both ends of the court if possible

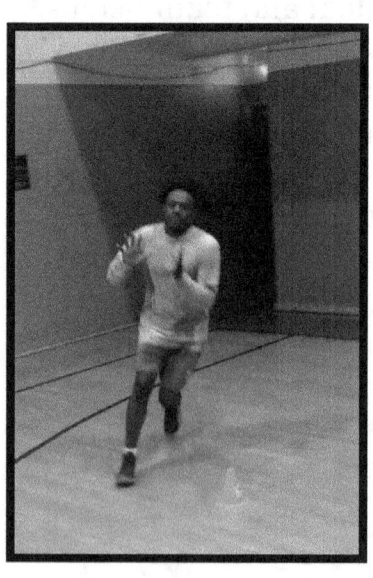 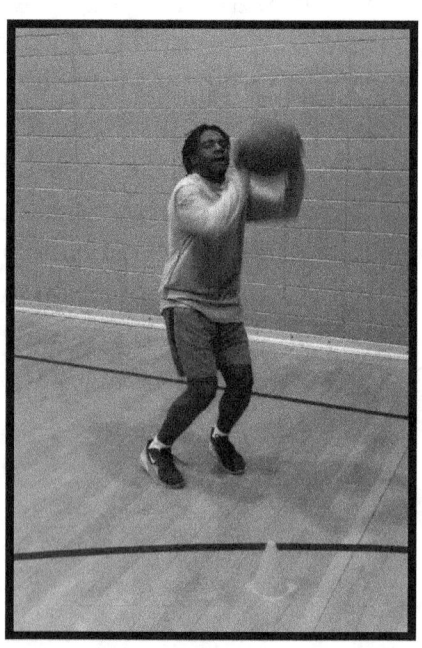

so that kids get to take more shots.] Every player has a basketball.

Players then take it in turns shooting with the aim to swish each shot through the net. The swish is important because we're trying to teach the kids how to shoot with enough arc on the shot.

After a player has taken a shot, they can either return to the end of the same line or rotate lines either clockwise or counter-clockwise.

21 Cones – Shooting Drill

All players are in two teams and each time a player hits a shot, they're awarded a cone for their team.

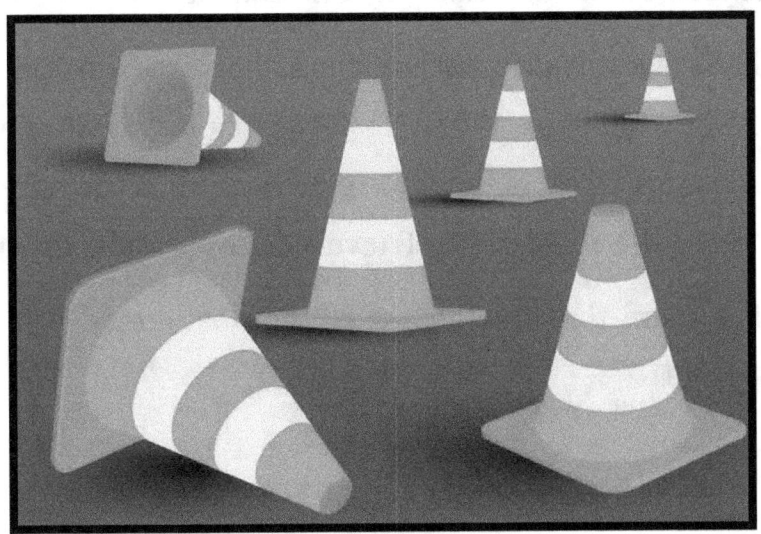

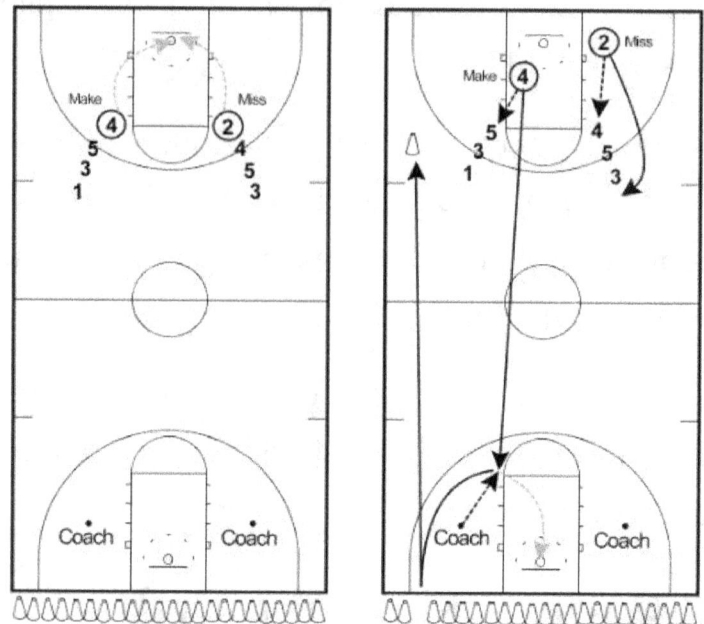

Place 21 cones on the baseline of one end of the court and then split your players up into two teams. Each team has only one basketball.

The two teams of players shoot from the designated spot. When a shot is made, the shooter is rewarded by being allowed to sprint to the other end of the court and retrieve a cone for their team.

The team that finishes with the most cones is the winner.

Pivot Shooting – Shooting Drill

This is a great drill that players will enjoy designed for incorporating footwork into a shooting drill.

Players perform a jump stop on receiving the pass from the coach, pivot around to square up to the basket, and then make a variety of scoring moves.

Players all start on the baseline in two lines. There are two coaches/parents at the top of the key. One in front of each line. Every player has a basketball.

Players will begin the drill by making a chest pass out to the coach in front of them. Immediately after making the chest pass, the player will explode to the free-throw line where the coach will pass the ball back to them.

After catching the basketball in a jump stop, the player must must pivot around using good technique and square up to the basket before shooting or attacking the ring.

Chase Down Layups – Shooting Drill

Chase down layups are used to teach players to finish layups at full speed and with pressure. Since youth basketball match-ups are normally decided by which team makes more layups, this is a drill that should be used often.

The drill begins with two lines of players down each end of the floor. One offensive line and one defensive line.

One basketball starts at the front of the offensive line at each end of the court.

The coach starts the drill by bringing the offensive player out from the baseline and gives them an advantage over the defender who always starts on the baseline. It's up to the coach's discretion how far in front the offensive player is.

We want the offensive player far enough in front that they must sprint while dribbling down the floor and then when they finish at the rim there is close defensive pressure behind them.

When they're both set up, the coach calls out 'GO' and both players sprint to the other end of the floor. The offensive player must try and finish at the rim and the defender must pressure the shot without fouling.

The pair then passes the basketball to the next player in line at their current end of the floor.

Pressure – Shooting Drill

Pressure is a simple and fun end-of-practice game that works on shooting free throws while under pressure.

All players form one line at the free throw line. The drill requires only one basketball.

Players take it in turns shooting free throws.

When a player makes a free throw, the person behind them is put under pressure. This means that if they miss, they're out of the game.

Once someone makes a shot, the pressure continues until someone misses. Once they do, there's no pressure until another shot is made.

This continues until there's a winner.

Dribbling Drills

Dribbling Lines – Dribbling Drill

This is a simple drill to teach the basics of dribbling to new players.

It's a good way to introduce new moves without overwhelming them and will also help to improve the technique of the movements players already know.

Every player has a basketball and lines up on the baseline. In a situation where there are more than 8 players, create two lines on the baseline instead of one.

The coach will instruct the players to use different dribbling movements to dribble up to either the half-court line or full court. The coach will explain the dribble movement to be performed first, and then say 'Go'.

Dribbling Drills

Here are a few that you can use:

- ✓ Right hand
- ✓ Left hand
- ✓ Two balls

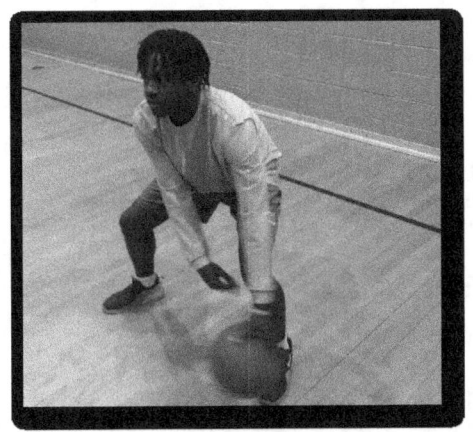

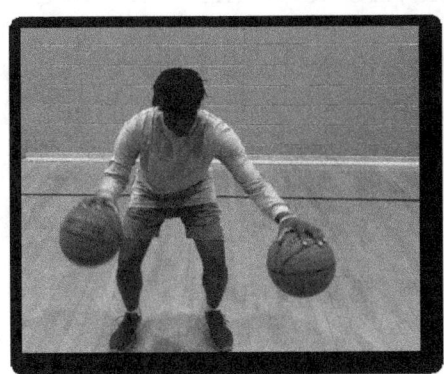
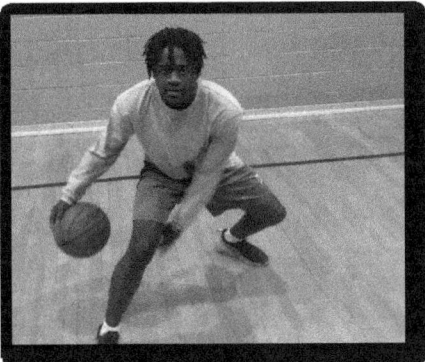

- ✓ Through-the-legs
- ✓ Dribble low
- ✓ Dribbling backwards

Dribble Knockout – Dribbling Drill

This drill works on ball-handling and protecting the dribble.

All players dribble around in a small area and the goal is to knock other players' basketball out of the area while keeping your own basketball alive.

The first thing the coach must do is determine the area the players will be dribbling in. This will depend on the number of players you have, but will usually be the three-point line or the 1/3 court line. All players must have a basketball.

On the coach's call, all players begin dribbling and attempt to knock each other's basketball out of the playing area. As more and more players get out, the coach must pause the game and make the playing area smaller. This continues until you have a winner.

Collision Dribbling – Dribbling Drill

Similar to dribble knockout except players are NOT allowed to hit the basketball of the other players away.

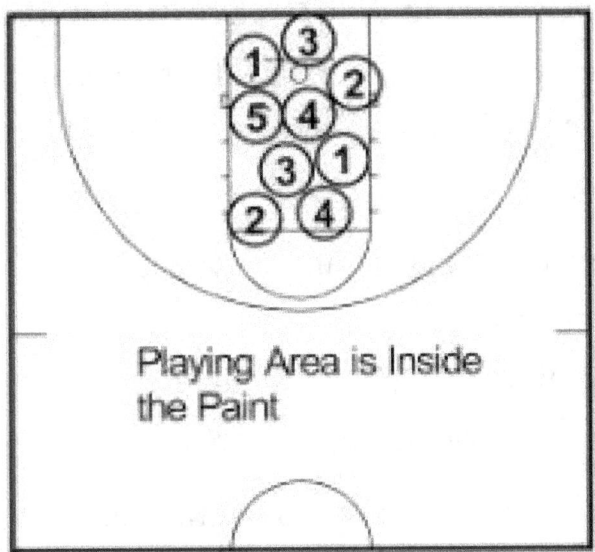

Instead, the aim of the drill is to navigate through and dodge all the other players using dribbling moves and by being creative with the dribble.

All players have a basketball and are in a small space determined by the coach.

On the coach's call, all players will start dribbling around each other in the small space aiming to keep their dribble under control. This drill will improve ball-handling because players must react to other players and can't predetermine their actions. It also forces all players to keep their heads up or they'll run into someone!

Scarecrow Tiggy – Dribbling Drill

Scarecrow Tiggy is a fun drill that involves everyone dribbling around trying to avoid two taggers.

Players love this drill and it's great for developing ball-handling skills. Every player starts with a basketball and begins in the half court except two players who will be the 'taggers'.

The taggers don't have a basketball and preferably are wearing different colored singlets so that other players can identify them.

The drill begins when the coach calls out 'GO'. The taggers then do their best to tag each player dribbling a basketball.

When a dribbler is tagged, they must stand in the place they were tagged with their legs wide and hold the ball on top of their head. They can be freed by other dribblers by rolling the basketball through their legs.

This game never has a winner unless the taggers happen to get everyone out at one time (this doesn't happen often). Every couple of minutes switch the taggers.

Dribble Tag – Dribbling Drill

Similar to Scarecrow Tiggy, except that all players start with a basketball (even the taggers) and when you're caught, you're out and must sit down on the side of the court.

This will depend on the amount of players you have. After that, select two players to be taggers and get everyone else to spread out around the court.

When the drill starts, the taggers attempt to tag as many dribblers as possible. When a dribbler is tagged, they are now out and must wait on the sideline for the rest of the players to be caught. This continues until there is one dribbler left and they are the winner.

Sharks and Minnows – Dribbling Drill

Sharks and Minnows is an amazing drill for youth practices.

The aim of the game is for the minnows (dribblers) to dribble from baseline to baseline without getting tagged by the sharks (taggers).

The drill starts with you selecting one or two 'sharks' who will be the taggers. Everyone else will start on the baseline and must have a basketball. These are the 'minnows'.

On the coach's call, the minnows must attempt to dribble to the other baseline without getting tagged by a shark.

If a shark does tag them, they must stand in the spot they were tagged, place the basketball between their feet, and are now scarecrows. If a minnow comes within reach of them, they can tag them to get them out. The last player alive, that hasn't been tagged, is the winner.

Passing Drills

Partner Passing – Passing Drill

Partner passing teaches the absolute basics of passing and allows your players to practice different types of passes and the correct technique.

A great drill for kids beginning to learn the game of basketball: Players get into pairs. Once the players are in pairs, they must stand on a line parallel from their partner [they should have one basketball between them].

The coach will explain which type of pass they want performed and then the players will pass back and fourth to each other. Every minute or so the coach can change the type of pass the players are performing or increase the distance they are apart if it's too easy.

Stationary Keepings Off – Passing Drill

This main goal of this drill is to teach the basics of spacing between players and also to teach decision making on the catch.

When players are young they constantly sprint towards the basketball. By keeping them stationary in this drill, we show them that it's easier to keep the ball away from the defense if we're spread apart.

Select one or two players to be the defenders and get the rest of your players to spread out in a small area like the three-point line. The team on offense will only need one basketball.

When the drill begins, the defenders will run around trying to steal the basketball from the offensive team. The defenders' goal is to get a deflection or a steal.

The offensive players must stay in one space and pass the ball around to each other keeping the basketball away from the defenders. After a minute or two, swap the defenders over.

Count Em' Up – Passing Drill

This drill is a more advanced version of the *Keepings Off* game. It works on getting open, denying the offensive player, and making smart passes to limit turnovers.

The first thing you need to do is split the kids up into two even teams. Preferably the teams are wearing different colors so that they can differentiate between each other during the drill. The drill involves only one basketaball.

The first thing that happens is that all players must match-up and stick to their individual opponent. The goal of the drill is to move around make a certain amount of passes set by the coach without the opposition deflecting the basketball or getting a steal. No dribbling or shooting allowed.

The amount of passes that must be made should be between 5 and 20 depending on age and experience. Players are allowed to move around wherever they want within the playing area.

If the defenders get a steal or deflect the basketball out of bounds, it becomes their ball and the offense and defense switch roles. For each time that a team successfully makes the certain number of passes, they get 1 point.

Continuous 3 on 2 – Passing Drill

This is one of the best drills for improving passing and decision making. As the name suggests, it's continuous 3 on 2. Having an extra player on offense means that there's always someone open as long as the offensive team keeps spaced apart.

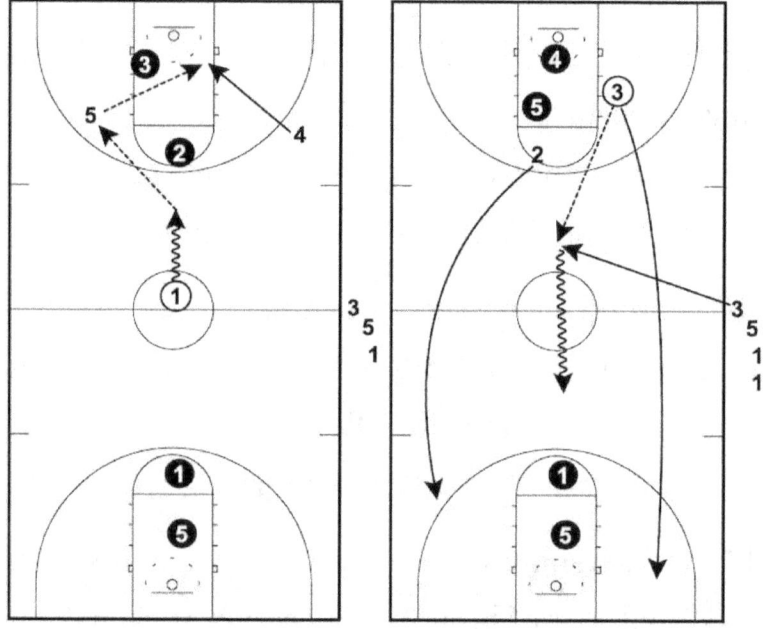

The drill starts with 3 offensive players in the middle of the court, 2 defenders in each half court, and the rest of the players standing out of bounds at the half court line. Only one basketball is needed for this drill.

The three offensive players attack two defenders at one end of the court and will either score or the defensive players will get the basketball.

Once the two defensive players get the basketball (either by steal, rebound, or because the offensive team scored), they outlet to the next player in line, at half way, who sprints in to help advance the ball.

The two defenders now become the offensive team and they get an extra player from the sideline to give them 3 players. They now attack towards the other end of the court 3 on 2.

As for the 3 previous offensive players, 2 of them become the next defenders and 1 of them joins the end of the out of bounds line. This process repeats for a set amount of time.

Footwork Drills

Four Corners – Footwork Drill

This is a great drill for working on jump stops, pivoting, and passing. It will allow the coach to teach the different kinds of pivots and is a drill the players enjoy doing.

The coach must first create a large square in the half-court by placing four cones an even distance apart. There must also be another cone or D-man in the exact middle of the square. You can see where I recommend placing these cones in the diagram.

Split your team up into four groups and send each group to a cone. The cones will be the starting position for each line. The person at the front of each line has a basketball.

The first thing the coach must do is tell the players which way they'll be passing (either right or left) and which kind of pivot they should use.

When the coach calls out 'Go', each player with a basketball dribbles in towards the middle cone, performs a jump stop a couple of feet away, pivots, and then passes to the next line before joining the end of it. The next player in the line that catches the basketball does not start until the coach has called out 'go' again.

Red Light, Green Light – Footwork Drill

This is a simple, but effective drill that will improve and allow you to teach jump stops and pivoting.

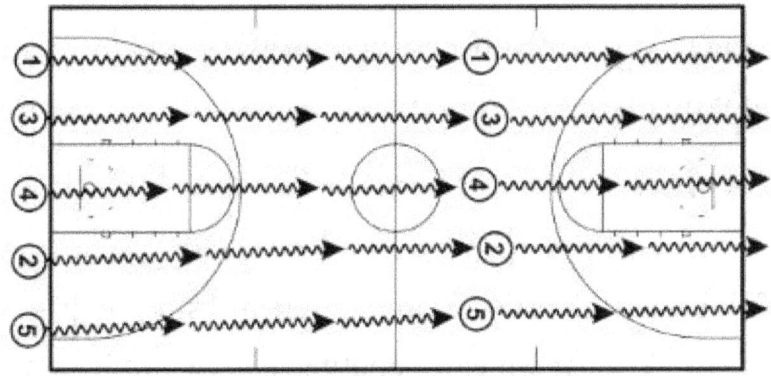

The drill starts with every player lined up along the baseline holding a basketball. If you have more than 10 players, it will be best to create two lines.

Everyone starts on the baseline in triple threat position. The coach will then lead the players up the court by calling out 'go' and 'stop'. On go, the players begin dribbling at a comfortable pace towards the opposite end of the court. When the coach says 'stop', the players must immediately perform a jump stop. This continues until the players reach the other end of the court.

Once your players are comfortable with the jump stops and are performing them correctly, you can make the drill more advanced by adding pivots. You can either say 'pivot' and allow them to pivot either way. Or you can be specific and say 'right foot pivot' or 'left foot pivot'.

Explode, Pivot, Pass – Footwork Drill

This drill focuses on basic footwork fundamentals. It's a really quick and simple drill to run. Your team can benefit greatly from it even if it's only run for 5 minutes.

Players get into groups of 2 or more (I prefer 3 players in each group-if possible). Each group has one basketball and should start in a straight line behind either the sideline, or the baseline.

The player starting with the basketball must begin the drill behind the line in triple threat stance. Their first action is to take two explosive dribbles out from the line and then perform a controlled jump stop.

After the jump stop, the player pivots 180 degrees until they're facing their group and makes a strong chest pass to the next person in line. They then jog to the end of the line.

The three main things coaches are looking at are:

- ✓ No traveling when exploding off the dribble.
- ✓ A controlled jump stop.
- ✓ A controlled pivot.

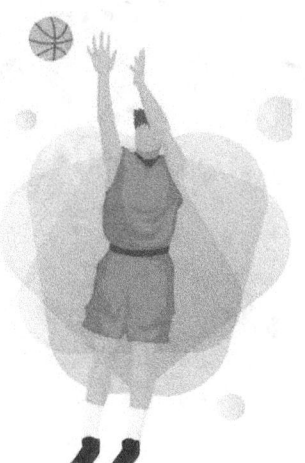
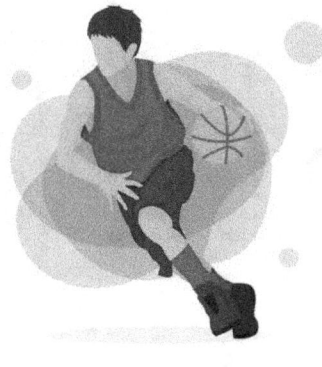

This process continues for a set amount of time.

Partner Drills

Try to have partners pair with same size and abilities, this will be more successful and rewarding. Partnering will also enhance the individual skills at passing and catching and are very quickly worked through so the chance of

getting bored is reduced. Partnering can be as fast or slow as the coach decides, and can follow any order that works well.

Close Out Drill

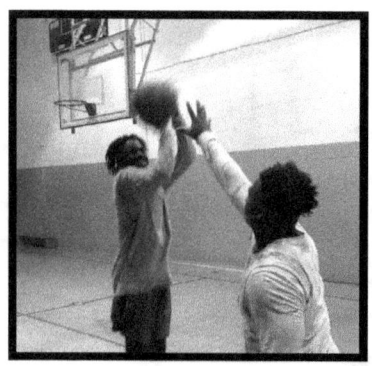 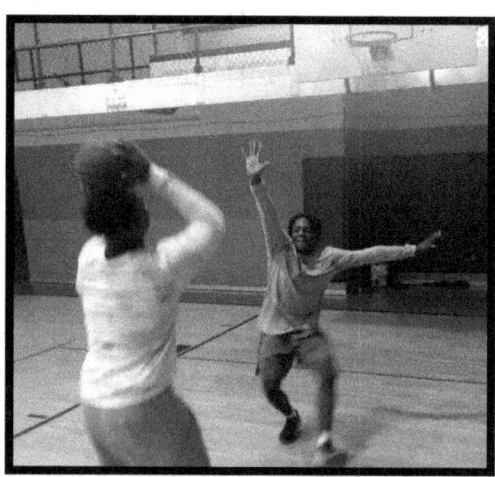

Stand about fifteen feet from each other, with one having a ball. First, roll the ball to the other person and then sprint and make a good close-out. Second, player one or two dribbles to whichever side he chooses. Then back to fifteen feet apart and the second player has the ball and repeats the drill. This can be repeated for a few minutes before moving on to another drill.

Box Out Drill

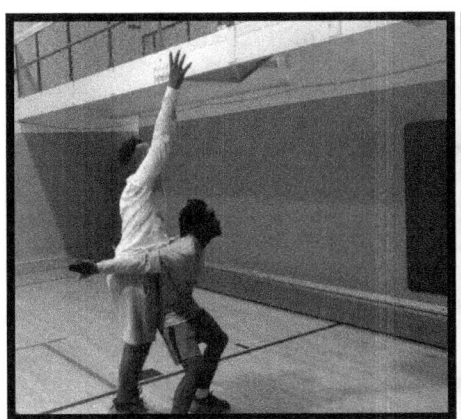 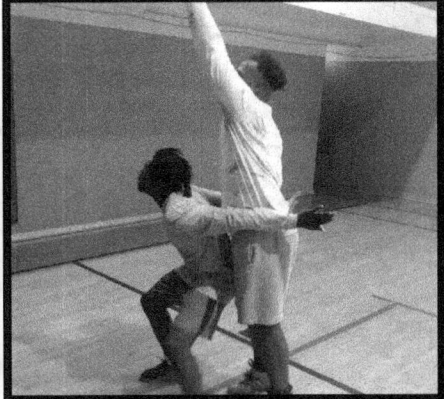

Players stand just a few feet from each other. Neither has a ball. The coach yells 'shot!' and the first player boxes out the second player by stepping up and making contact. Normally this is done with a forearm, followed by a quick pivot with feet wide and elbows out. At the coaches second call of 'shot!' the second player boxes out the first. Practice for a few minutes and then move on.

One- on- One Drill

Using both ends of the court, the player with the ball starts at the top and attempts to move or shoot an outside shot. The defender needs to stop the offense and get the rebound. Offense will then be awarded one point each for: a basket made, an offensive rebound, or if the defender fouls. There are no second shots here and each player must keep track of their own score. You should play up to five sets and the loser gets to do 5 – 10 push-ups.

Elbow Shooting

First player has the ball. Second player starts at his left elbow, then fakes left and cuts to the right. First player then passes to second player. Second player squares up and then takes a shot. Switch roles and repeat. You can do this for as many sets as you can, getting up to 40 shots for each player.

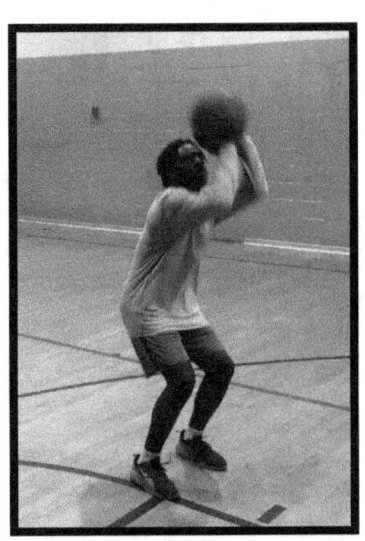

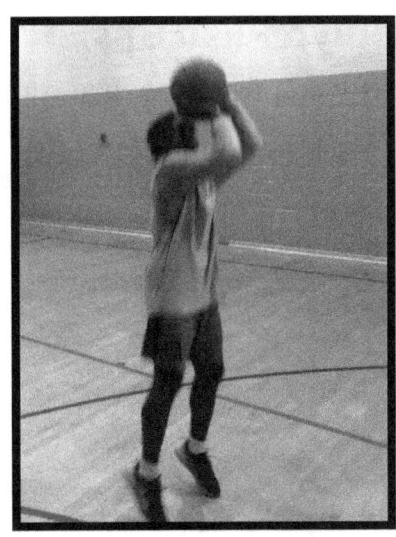

Strength and Conditioning Drills

The off season is the time when these skills and drills may be put into place. Players need to be strong enough to withstand contact, yet supple and quick enough to change direction in an instant. Off season is the perfect time to work on getting strong, both mentally and physically in order to play the game. Pre-season training for players is beneficial.

Plyo Push Ups

Plyo push-ups are done in a regular push up position, but with the ball between both hands. Lower yourself halfway to the ground and then

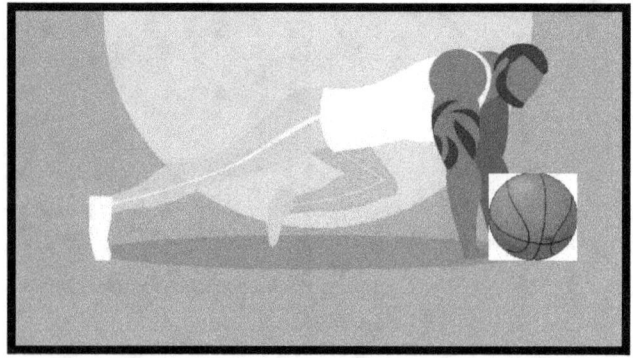

violently explode upwards off the floor to catch and land on the ball on the ground. Hold in this position for a second. Push up and off and replace hands on the floor.

Medicine Ball Throws

You should be facing a wall, with the ball in both hands, at chest height in front of you. As hard as you can, hurl the ball at the wall and be sure to catch it again as it bounces. Repeat for either set number of repetitions or selected time frame.

Medicine Ball Rotation Throws

Have your feet shoulder-width apart and face the wall sideways. With both hands holding the ball and arms slightly bent, swing the ball over your hip and against the wall. Keep your hands at the ready to catch the ball as it comes back at you. Make sure to swap sides so both sides are worked.

Medicine Ball Slams

Have your feet shoulder-width apart and the ball tucked behind your head. As hard as you can, slam the ball into the ground, squat down and pick up again. Repeat for any length of time or desired amount of repetitions.

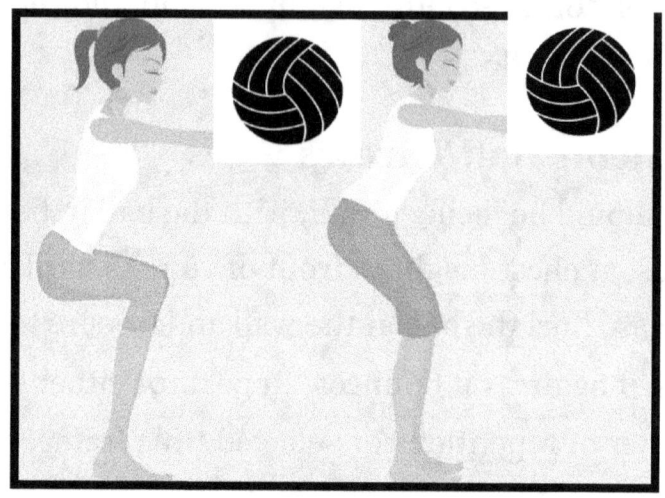

Medicine Ball Squat Throws

Have feet shoulder with apart and the ball at chest height. Quickly squat down to parallel position then jump straight up as fast as you can, pushing the ball above your head as high as you can reach. Let the ball drop, then pick it up and repeat again for a length of time or reps.

Cool Down Drills

After a basketball workout, it is really important that the body slowly returns to normal. It is vital to have a good cool down routine ,that includes stretches, to prevent injury. The aim of the cool down is to have the heart rate gradually return to normal, reduce the waste product lactose, and to reduce the risk of sore muscles.

Walking Without Shoes on

Get those basketball shoes off and walk around with no socks on. Focus on feeling every part of your feet from your heels right up to your toes

Practice Good Form

Stand in a relaxed position with feet shoulder width apart and arms to your sides. Slowly lift your shoulders up towards your ears, feel as if you are moving them backwards and then downwards to a relaxed position. Take a deep breath and repeat again

Single Knee Cross

Lie on a mat on a soft floor with hands at sides and both knees bent, feet on the floor. Lift one foot and place on other knee and gently push down on the lifted knee to stretch hips. A good basketball knee pad will come in handy here.

Hold for 20 seconds and then change and do the other side.

Ankle Rotations

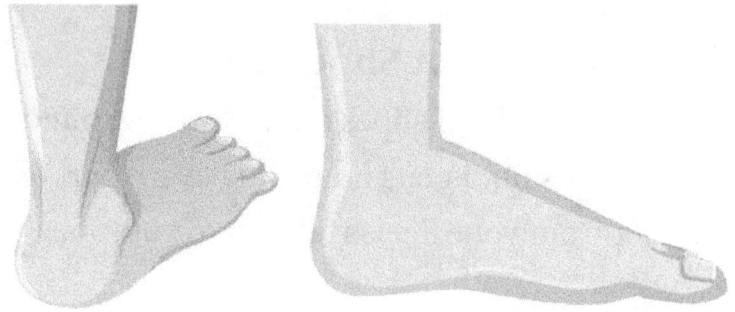

Sit on a chair and lift one leg at a time. Gently rotate ankles one way and then the other direction. Do this nice and slowly. Now, change and do the other ankle.

Shoulders and Neck

This should be done slowly and smoothly. Stand comfortably and hang arms at sides. Look right and hold, then turn head left and hold. Then return to the front. Now turn slightly to the right and look down to the floor. You will feel your neck muscle stretch. Hold for a bit then turn to the other side and repeat.

Calves

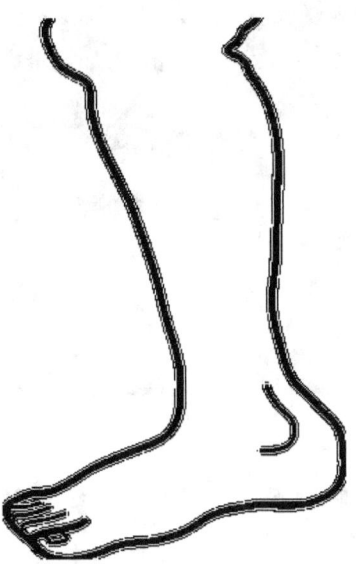

Find a step where you can support yourself. Stand on the step with your heels off the back and slowly lower your heels as far as is comfortable. Then – again slowly – raise up on your toes until you are as high as you can. Hold again, then relax.

Defensive Drills

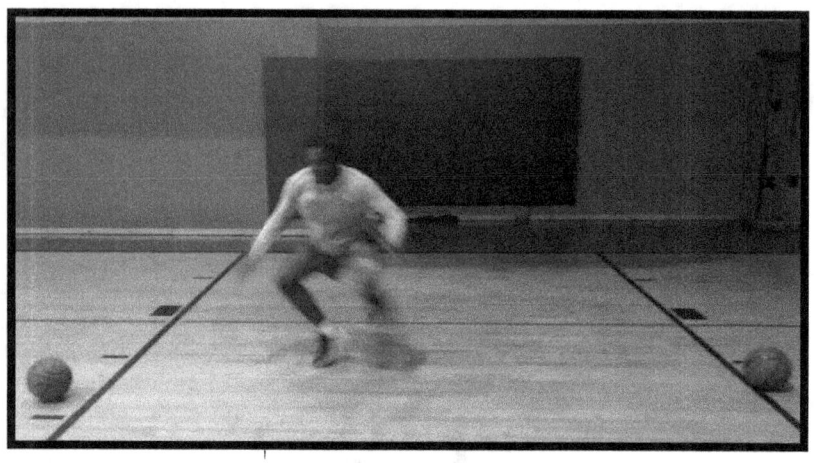

Defensive Mirrors – Defense Drill

This is a fun drill for working on defensive footwork.

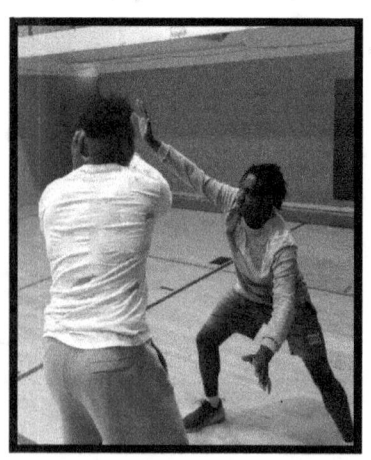
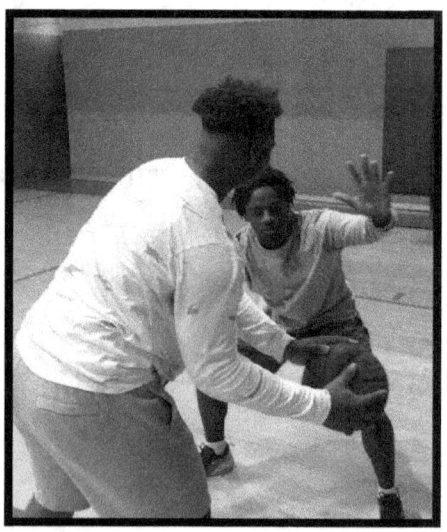

More Defensive Drills

The drill requires players to mimic their partner's movements which is great for developing reactions while working on defensive footwork.

The only problem with this drill is that only two people can go at once so if you have a large group it might not be appropriate.

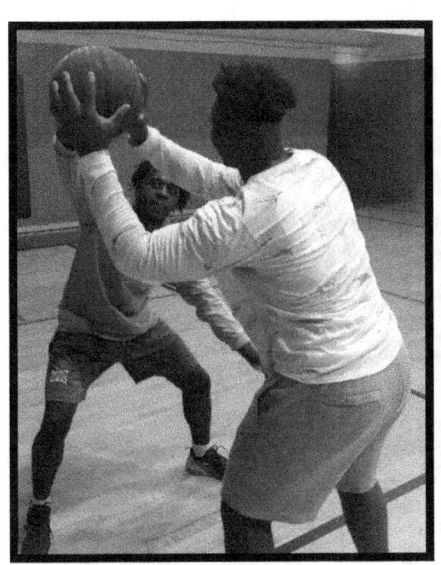
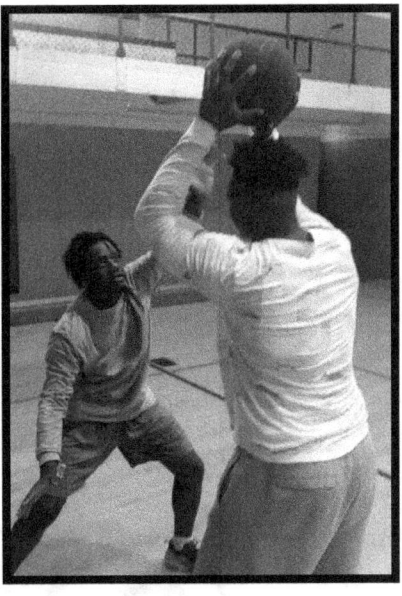

Everyone starts by finding a partner and standing in pairs behind the baseline. If you have another coach, it's best to use both ends of the court.

For this example, we'll use the parallel lines of the key, but if you have two other parallel lines on your home court, you can use them too.

The first pair comes out and sets themselves up directly opposite each other on the two parallel lines of the key.

The coach then assigns one of them the offensive player and the drill begins immediately.

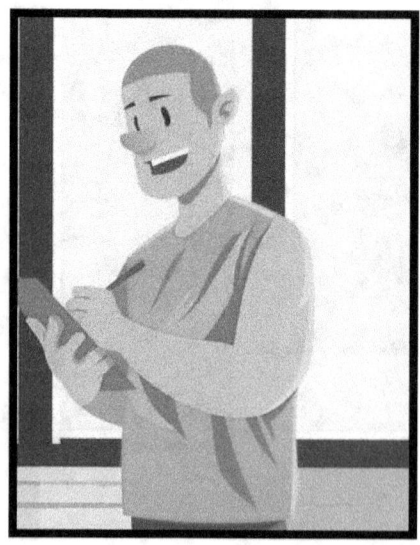

The goal of the defensive player is to stay directly in line with the offensive player. The offensive player must work hard to try and separate themselves from being in line with the defender by sliding up and down the line of the key.

After 15 seconds, the coach calls out 'switch' and the two players swap roles. After 30 seconds they step behind the baseline and two new players come in.

Defensive Specialist – Defense Drill

Defensive Specialist is a continuous drill that works on the different defensive movements players will make on defense including closeouts, defensive sliding, back-pedalling, and sprinting.

Since it's hard to explain where the cones and movements are by writing, I encourage you to take a look at the image associated with this drill for better comprehension. You will require four D-men or cones for this drill. All players begin in a straight line on the baseline.

All players line up in a straight line on the baseline. Players perform this defensive course one-by-one.

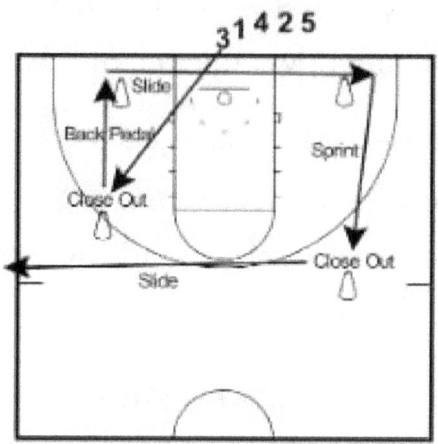

The first movement is a sprint and then close out to the cone in front. The player then back-pedals around a cone directly behind them, and then slides across to the other side of the court.

When the first defender slides past the line, that triggers the next player in line to start the drill.

When the first defender has slid around the cone on the other side of the court, they again sprint to close out, and then once again slide to the opposite side of the court before returning to the end of the line Depending on the number of players you have, run this drill for 3 – 5 minutes.

One-on-One – Defense Drill

One-on-One drills are amazing and can teach both defense and offense.

By playing one-on-one, we're forcing the on-ball defender to have to 'guard their yard'. There's no help defense coming. They're on their own and must stay in front and challenge the shot.

This drill starts with two players at the free-throw line or top of the key depending on age and experience.

The defensive player starts with the basketball. The other players wait behind them near half-way. Use both ends of the basketball court if you have two coaches so that players get to play more often.

To start the drill, the defender hands the basketball to the offensive player. By handing the basketball to the offensive player, it ensures that the defender is challenging themselves by starting up close to the offensive player instead of standing back playing lazy defense. The offensive player then has a maximum of 2 or 3 dribbles to attack the ring and get a clear shot.

Offensively, this drill teaches players not to waste their dribble and teaches them how to attack a defender one-on-one. Defensively, players will learn how to keep an offensive player in front of them and challenge every shot.

After either a make or a miss, a new offensive player comes in, the previous offensive player switches to defense, and the previous defender joins the end of the line.

Zig-Zag Slides – Defensive Drill

Zig-zag slides are a great drill for a beginning team. The two most important lessons this drill teaches are: how to defensive slide properly and how to drop step when playing defense.

The drill begins with all players on the baseline lining up on one of the corners. No player should have a basketball.

The first player will defensive slide from the corner to the high post and perform a 90-degree drop step so that they are now sliding back to the opposite sideline.

This process of sliding from one side to the other and drop stepping continues until the player reaches the opposite baseline. They come back down the opposite side of the court using the same principles.

Fun Drills
War – Fun Drill
War is a great drill to incorporate fun small-sided games into your practices. It's a series of small-sided games between two teams that can be played in both the full-court and half-court. This is always a favorite drill no matter what level of coaching.

The drill is set up by splitting your group into two teams and lining each half up along opposite sidelines.

For example, let's say there are 12 players total and 6 players on each team. You will give individual players on each team a number from 1 – 6.

The drill requires one basketball and it always starts with the coach.

The drill begins with the coach throwing a basketball out into the middle of the court and calling out a few numbers between 1 and 6.

If the coach wants to play games of 3 on 3, they might call out "1, 4, and 5!" If this happens, numbers 1, 4, and 5 from both teams come out and play a game of 3 on 3 until a score occurs. The coach can play games with any number of players from 1 on 1 to 6 on 6.

Golden Child – Fun Drill

Golden child is another fun game that kids will end up begging you to let them play each practice.

It involves splitting up into two teams, a shooting team and a dribbling team, and then the dribbling teams must run around the half-court one-by-one while the shooters try and get them out.

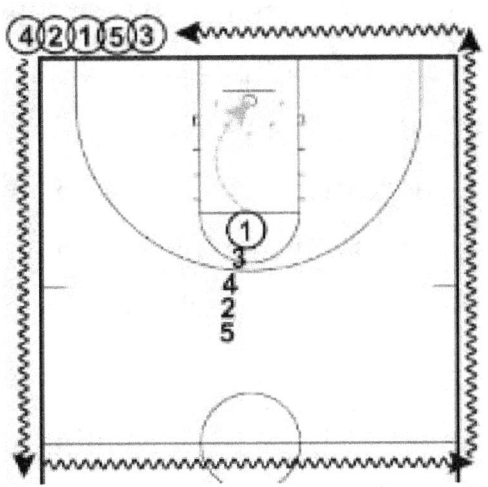

The first step is to split your group up into two similarly even teams. The dribbling team must all have a basketball and they should be lined up at one of the corners of the baseline.

The shooting team will have one or two basketballs and will be lined up around the free-throw line or closer depending on age and skill.

The drill begins with the coach calling out 'Go!' which triggers both teams to start.

For the dribblers, the goal of the game is to make as many home runs as they can. A home run is when a dribbler makes it all the way around the outside of the half court and back to the line.

The shooters must attempt to get them out by making a shot. If a shot is made the shooters must call out 'STOP' and the current dribbler must freeze. The next dribbler can begin immediately when this happens. If they make it home, they get one run and can join the end of the line to run again.

This continues until all the dribbling players are out and then the teams switch roles. The team with the most amount of runs at the end of the game wins.

Elimination – Fun Drill

The goal of the game is to make your shot before the person behind you makes their shot. The first shot must always be from the free throw line, but after that can be from anywhere on the floor.

All players line up in a straight line behind the free throw line. The first two players in line have a basketball.

The drill begins with the first person in line taking a shot. If they make it, they quickly rebound their ball and throw it to the next person in line. If they miss, they must rebound the ball and score as quickly as possible.

As soon as the first player has shot, the second player can begin.

If the player behind scores before the player in front, the player in front is out. The drill continues until there is one person left and they are crowned the winner.

Small-Sided Games – Fun Drill

Do kids love anything more than playing a real game of basketball? Depending on the number of players you have, I believe 3 on 3 or 4 on 4 are the best small-sided games to use.

Use both halves of the court and create small-sided games depending on the number of players you have.

Tell each team they must advance the ball to either half-court or the third line of the court if you have one. Each game needs one basketball.

Start the game and play! Make adjustments and team changes when you need to, but I recommend trying not to interrupt too much. Let the players learn from their own mistakes through experience.

Game-Winner – Fun Game

This drill is an awesome way to finish practice on a high note. Each time I run this drill, the players end up leaving practice with a smile on their faces.

All it is is one long-distance shot where, if made, the shooter wins some kind of prize or award.

Depending on the age of your team, select a distance away from the basket that is outside of their comfortable shooting range, but close enough that the kids can still throw/shoot the basketball and there's a chance it will go in. All you need is one basketball for this drill.

For this example, we'll say that distance is the half-way line. Get all the players in one line at half-way and they each take a single shot. The players that makes the shot receives a reward from the coach. This could be anything from a small prize to being the leader of warm-ups the following week.

Drills Every Basketball Player Should Master

For the love of the game. That's why anyone should play any sport, right? Because you love it. And when you love something, you should ponder over why it's so important to you and how you can make it even better. Basketball is one of those sports that a player can get by on his or her natural abilities, but they cannot excel without practicing the skills necessary to be outstanding.

While a lot of practice is physical, the majority of it is mental- preparing for situations which may occur in real games, While you may not be able to foresee when or how they will exactly occur, you can do your best to be as ready for them as possible. Drills to help you take the element of surprise out and put the element of reaction in are what separates those "just getting" by from those wanting to master the game they love. Grab a couple of teammates, some basketballs and a trash can because, no matter your age, these are drills every player should master.

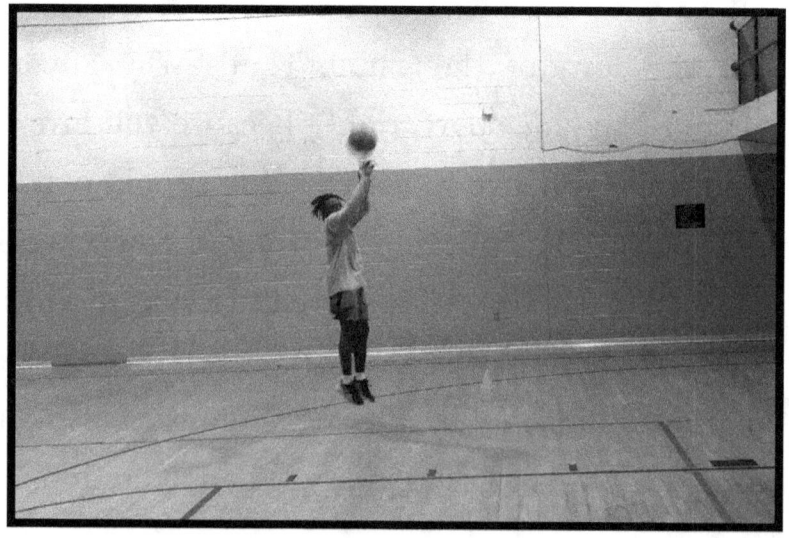

Full Speed Shooting

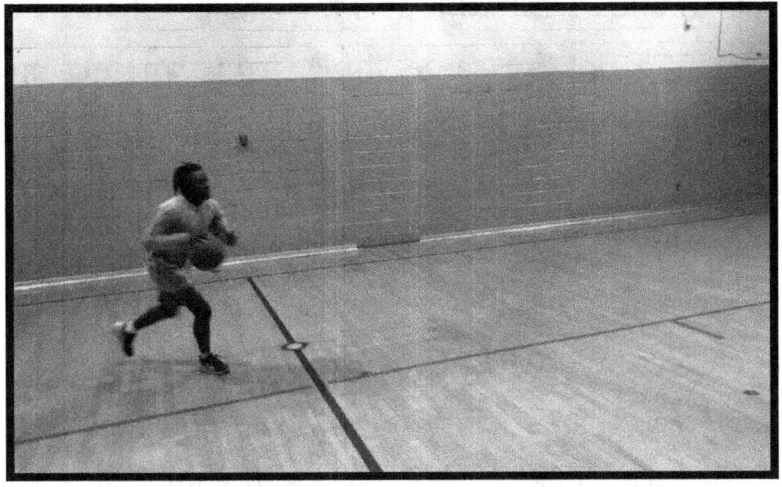

Warming up and shooting around the top of the key is a good way to get loose and help you visualize the ball going into the basket as you shoot. But you won't have the luxury of nonchalantly moseying around the arch with no defender and no sense of urgency. Full speed shooting teaches you to shoot while on the run and have a need to stop-and-pop and it teaches you the necessary energy needed to shootwhen you are beginning to get tired. Run in full speed from half-court to anywhere on or right inside the arch to shoot. After your shot, backpedal to half court and do the same thing. You can mix-up whether it's stop-and-pop or one dribble pull up, but you must make 20 shots before you can stop. This may seem easy when you start off and get that first 10, but then your legs don't give you as much lift and your arms aren't giving you the consistent stroke you're needing to complete the task. Learn to perfect this drill and your ability to push through that last minute in the fourth quarter, when everyone else is dog tired, will be the difference between a body on the floor and a game-changer.

Cutt off (1 on 1 Closeouts)

One-on-one is a lost art. Now it's merely a game of wonderment with no applicable real-game situations. Too much dribbling. Ridiculous shots that can only be taken in a one-on-one matchup. One-on-one via "Cutt off" with closeouts is your best real-game experience with rules implemented to challenge the scorer and the defender. This isn't your normal "check ball." Multiple players take turns rolling the ball from under the hoop to the offensive player at the top of the key and closeout, forcing the offense to go one way or the other and forcing the defender to react quickly. Allow only two dribbles per possession (three max) because if it takes you more than that to get from the top of the key to the hoop, you aren't taking a direct path and another defender is likely to come into play in a real game. You score, you stay on offense. You get scored on, back of the line and let the next defender have a crack at it until the defense gets a stop and then goes to offense. First player to 10 wins. This is as "real game" as it gets when you don't have 10 players to form two teams.

Defensive Lane Slides

Lane slides are one of the simplest drills to do, but one of the hardest to perfect. And that's really only because it's damn near impossible to perfect the defensive slide, especially in real-game

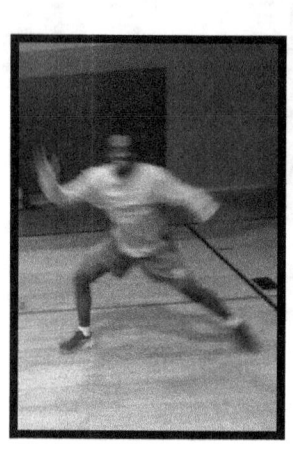 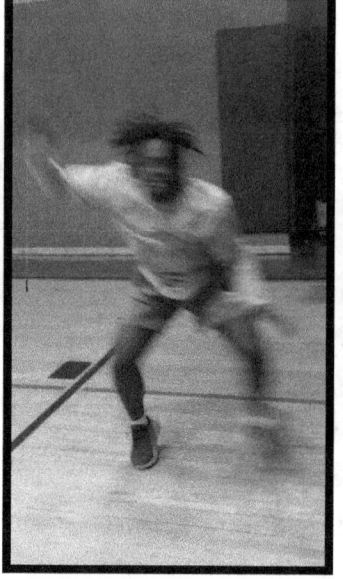 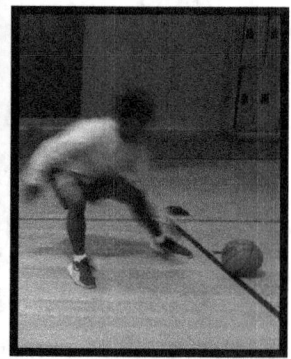

Two Ball Passing

Passing is one of the most fundamental components of basketball - even if there are players on your team who refuse to learn it. Learning how to give a basic chest or bounce pass should be an elementary procedure but taking it to the next level and throwing in other forms of passing and adding in an additional ball is another drill that tests your concentration. One player bounce passes while the other simultaneously chest passes, catches and repeats. You can throw in variables of speed, types of bounce/chest passes (one player gives a low-post at one's side to the left while the other gives the same pass to the right) that force you to learn the correct way to pass from every angle and direction.

Curl, Fade, Cut

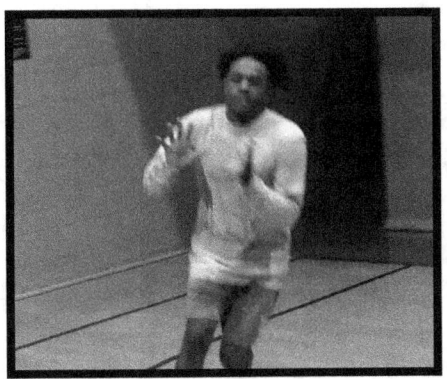

A great way to know if a player is smart or not is if they can read how a defender is guarding them off of a screen. There should only be three options a decent defender is giving the offense coming off of a screen. If the defender is following behind the offense, you should curl.

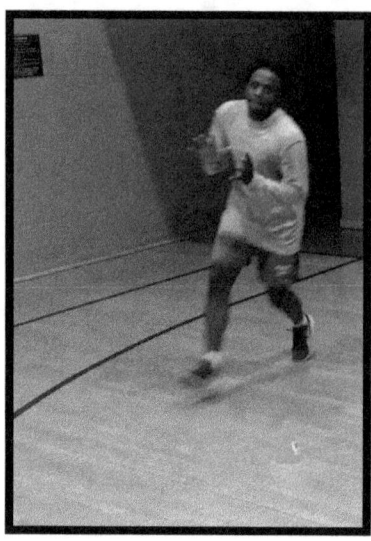 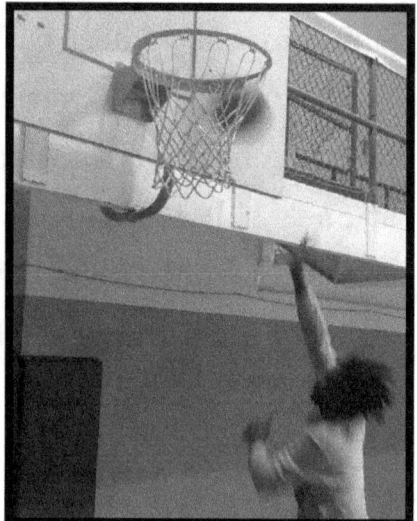

If he goes over top of the screen but is still in good position, you fade. If he's completely overplaying and gambling on a potential pass, give them the ol' backdoor cut for a layup. That's only half of it though, as you must learn how to shoot off of these three moves. Have the defender mix up their defense coming off of a screen (which can be a trashcan) while the offense determines the best course of action to get the best possible shot.

Two-Ball Dribbling

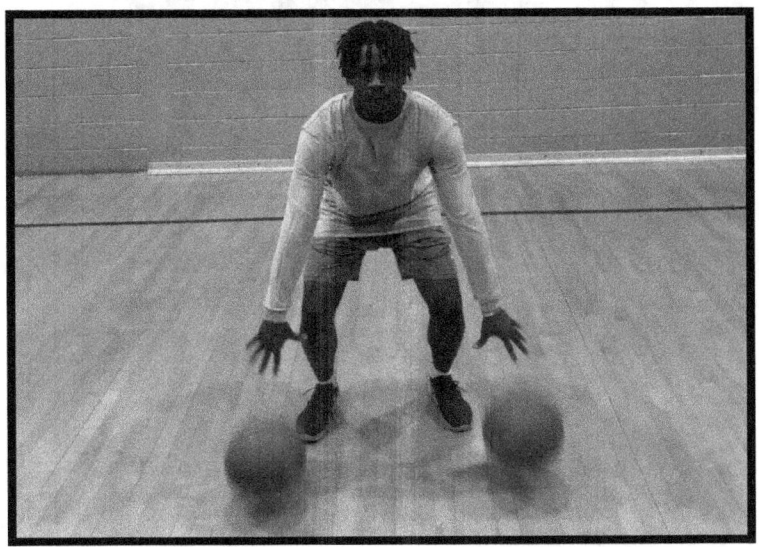

Everyone needs to dribble the ball. Everyone needs to be able to dribble the ball, with both hands, to be successful. While one-ball dribbling drills allow you to concentrate on perfecting your handle with one hand, two balls force you to concentrate, even with the distraction of using both hands at once.

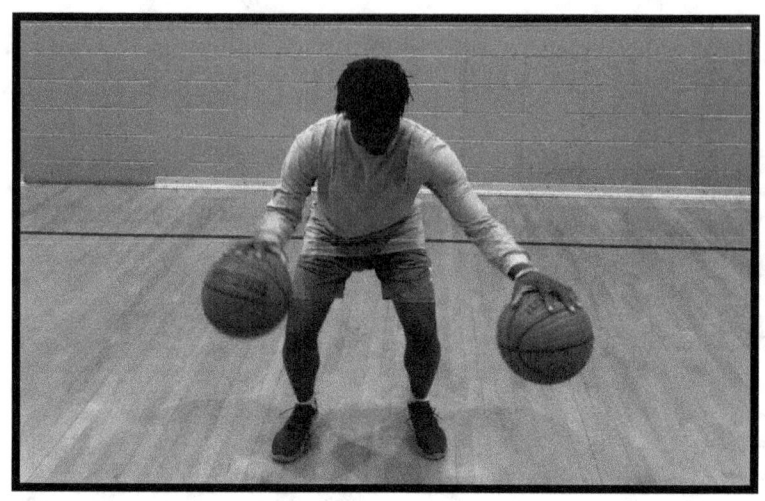

There are a variety of drills you can do within this one, usually starting from stationary simultaneous dribbling, then moving to a variation of stationary and moving drills from alternating dribbles to uneven dribbles (one ball bouncing high, one ball staying low.) All while keeping your head up. You must learn where the ball should be at all times without looking at it so you can concentrate on other in-game decisions you'll need to make.

Mikan/Reverse Mikan

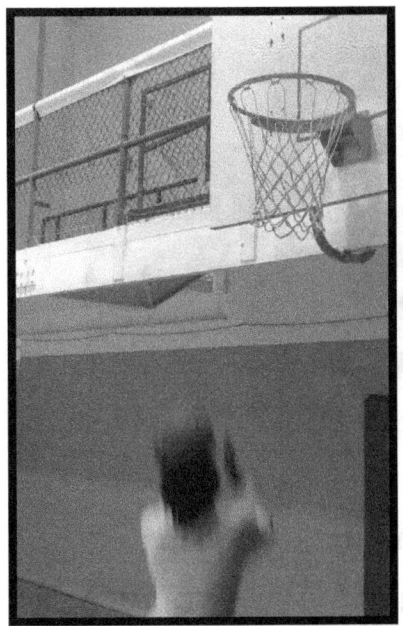
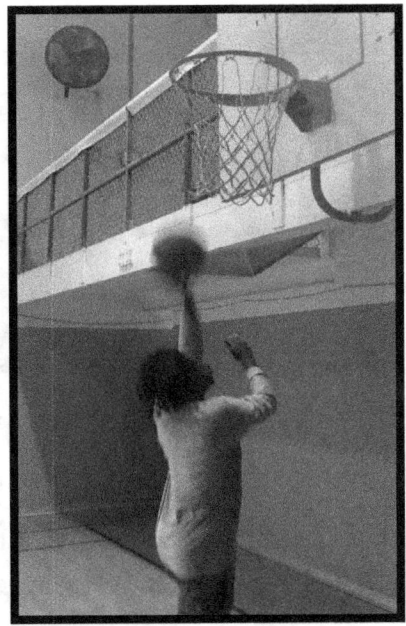

Thanks to one of the fore-fathers of basketball, George Mikan, we have one of the greatest warm-up drills ever. The Mikan drill involves shooting close-up layups off one foot, while alternating from one side of the basket to the other in a fluid motion. While it may look easy, there are governing rules.

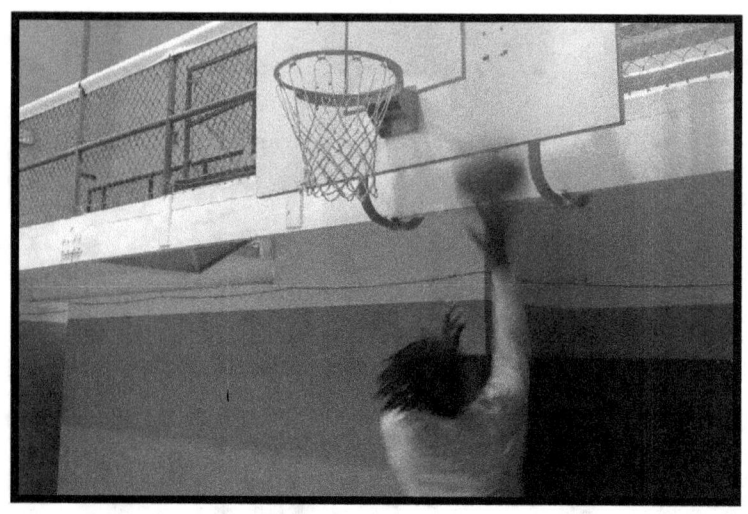

You must keep the ball above your shoulders, which is the easiest rule to break because your natural inclination when jumping is to bring your arms, and the ball, down so you have more propulsion when going up. By keeping the ball above your head, you're keeping it closer to the basket, allowing you to get to the basket quicker. Another rule is that, once you miss, you have to start your count over. You could start easy and make 10 in a row from each side of the basket, but once it's become a regular warmup, try and make 25 in a row. Go for 50 if you're ambitious. Oh, and then you have to do the same thing, but with reverse layups. Muscle memory and discipline, which are the results of this drill, can lead to easy buckets under the hoop.

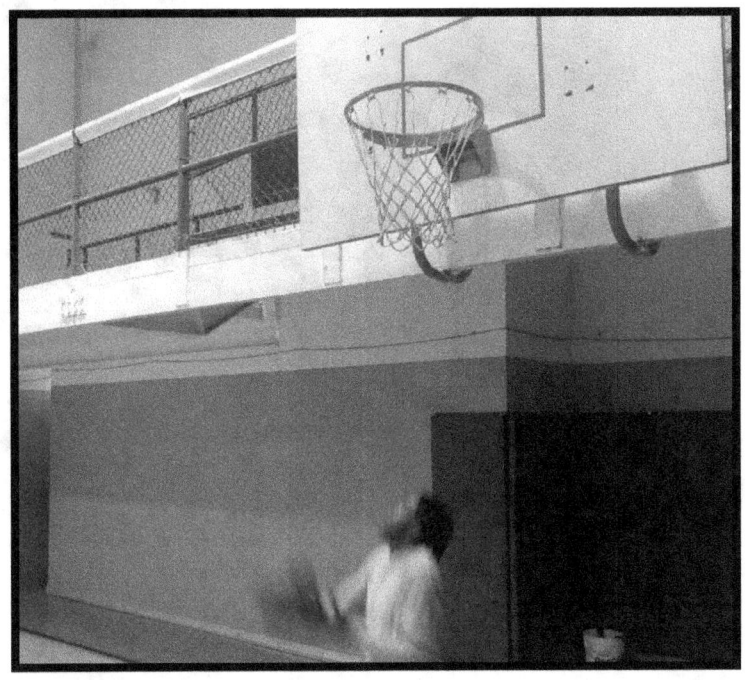

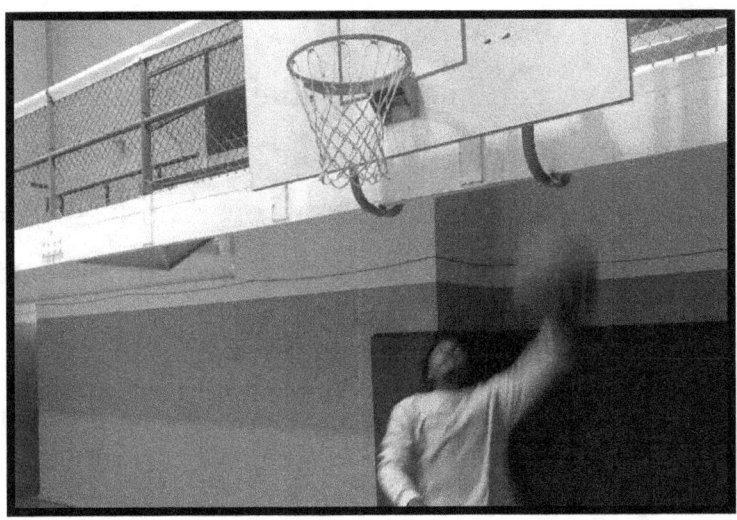

Post "Crab" Dribble Moves

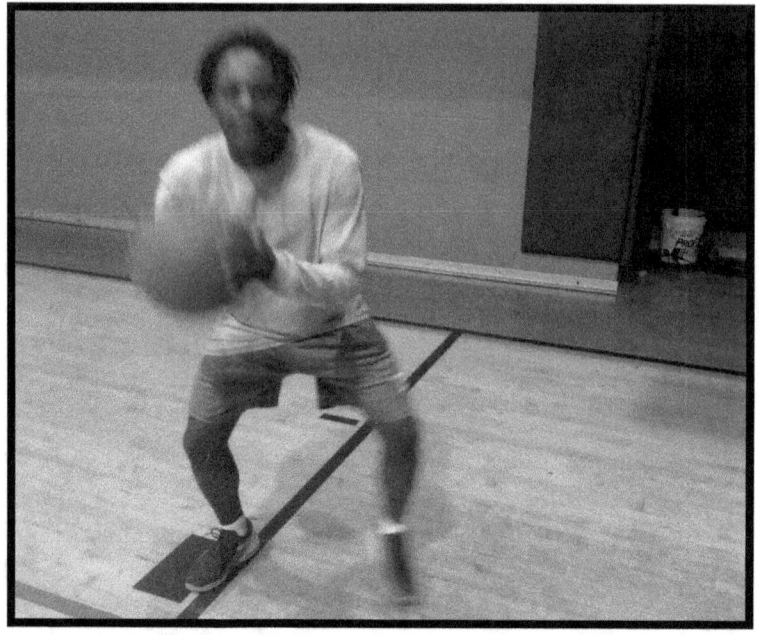

Big men need love too, right? They provide that body in the lane who can be a terror on defense and a force to be reckoned with on offense, but if they have soft moves in the post, guess whose touches will slowly dwindle? This move teaches you to make strong moves over both shoulders with the one dribble every big man should perfect; the post-crab dribble. You know, that two-handed power dribble you take before you go up off two-feet and try to jam it on someone?

The passer feeds the ball to the big man in the post and, based on which hip their defender is playing closest to, they give one low, but strong crab dribble to the opposite side. Sometimes that will be straight to the basket for a layup. Once you've gone both directions, an added bonus would be to practice the same move but with a pump-fake, un-and-under move. Remember; strong crab dribble and strong finish

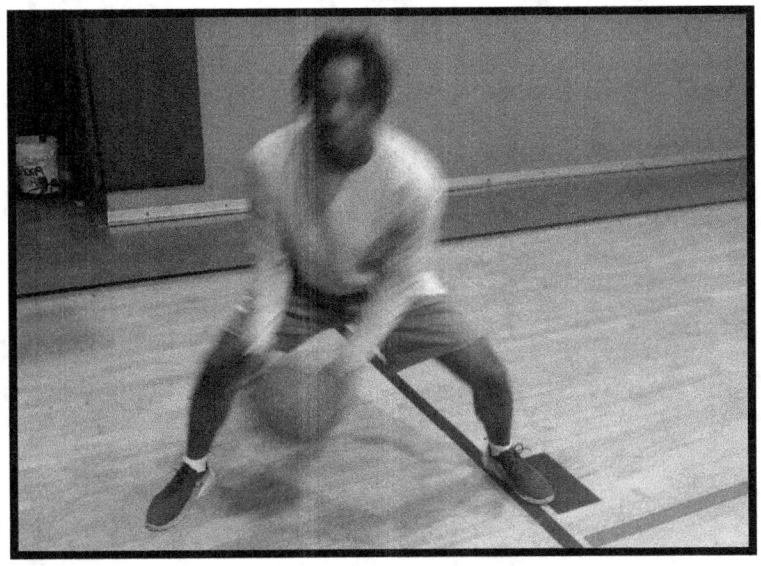

from a low position will ensure you get fed in the post as much as you can take.

Full Speed Dribbling

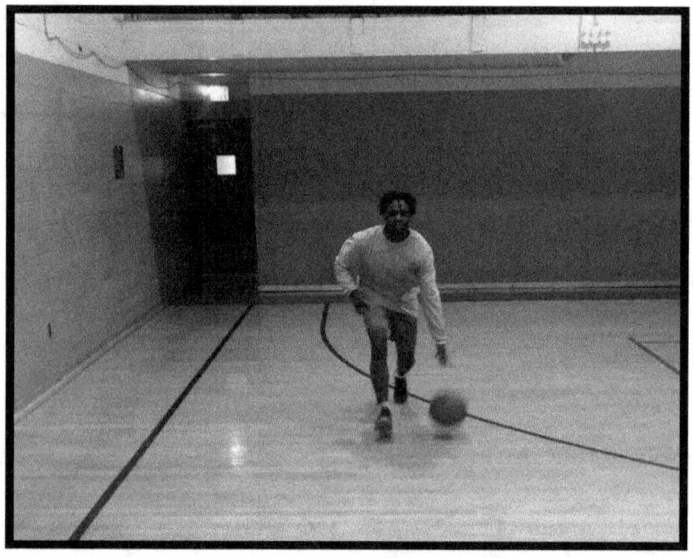

Shooting off the dribble is difficult. It can be trained and engrained into our games, but it's hard to perfect. Coming up the court full speed and making a move on a defender to shoot is near impossible to perfect, but once you get this drill into your workout, it will at least feel like a natural way of doing things. All this drill takes is a basketball and a trash can as a defender.

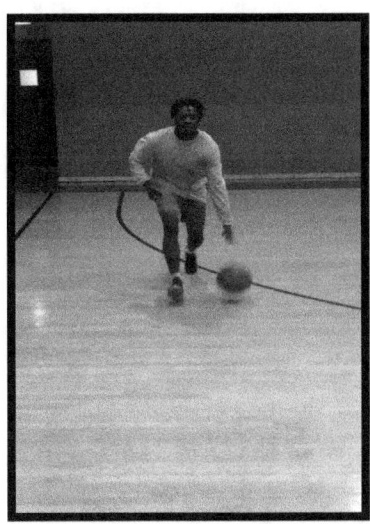 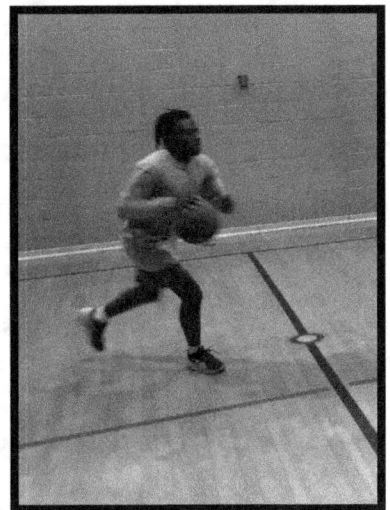

Learning to run full speed at something and stopping to make a move one way or another, while tough for an offensive player to do right, is even tougher for a defender to defend. Switch up the move; crossover, in-and-out, even a spin every once in a while (with caution!) will allow you to make a split decision as you come at the defender, forcing them to make a decision in even shorter time. After the move, you can give a strong move to the whole with no more than two additional dribbles. Learning to pull up off of it gives you a dimension to your game that coaches go gaga over. In-between game (outside the lane, but inside the 3-point arch) is a precise commodity as a basketball player. All you have to do is look at Michael Jordan to understand this.

Muscle Memory Shooting

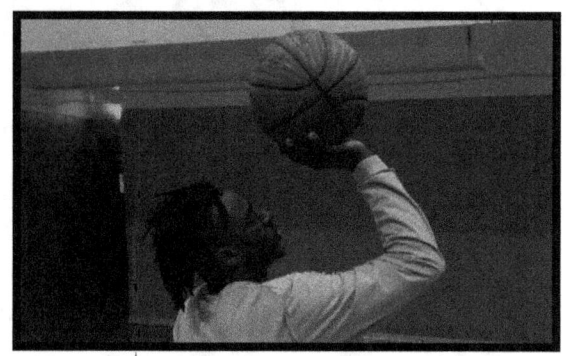

You walk in the gym and you stretch. What should be the next thing you do? It isn't take a dribble. It isn't a few laps. It should be muscle memory shooting. One-handed shots, starting at as close of range as possible and progressively moving out, keeping a rhythm as the ball drops through the hoop then go through the motion again. No matter the case, they've perfected whatever motion they shoot in because of muscle memory and this drill is your introduction to it.

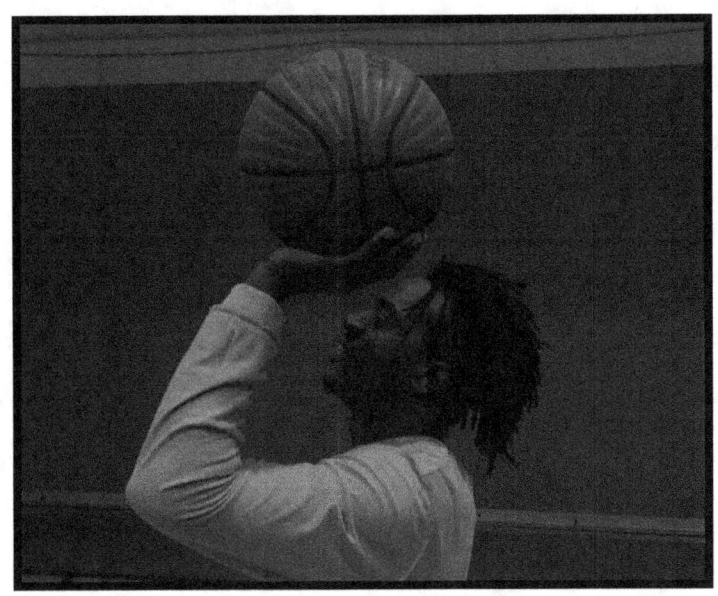

Eating Right

Basketball is an intermittent, high-intensity sport requiring both physical agility and mental acuity. Energy demands during the basketball season are

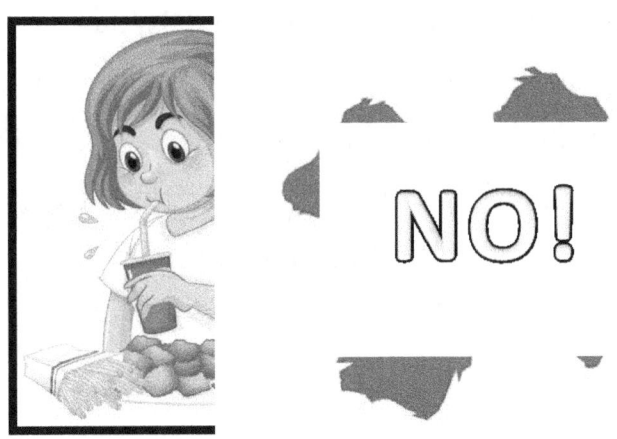

substantial and may be even higher during off-season training.

Choosing foods that will provide the energy to support competition and training is essential and can also be quite challenging. Unlike high-level college or professional basketball players who have the means and opportunity to eat a proper diet, smaller-school college players, high school athletes, and younger players have variable access to resources.

The energy requirements of high-school basketball players can be considerable. In a recent study by Silva et al, energy expenditure in elite high-school-aged female and male basketball players during the season was measured to be over 3,500 and 4,600 kcals/day, respectively. Although total energy intake is important to counteract weight loss during the season, the source of the calories is critical to provide the muscle with the right type of fuel.

Carbohydrates

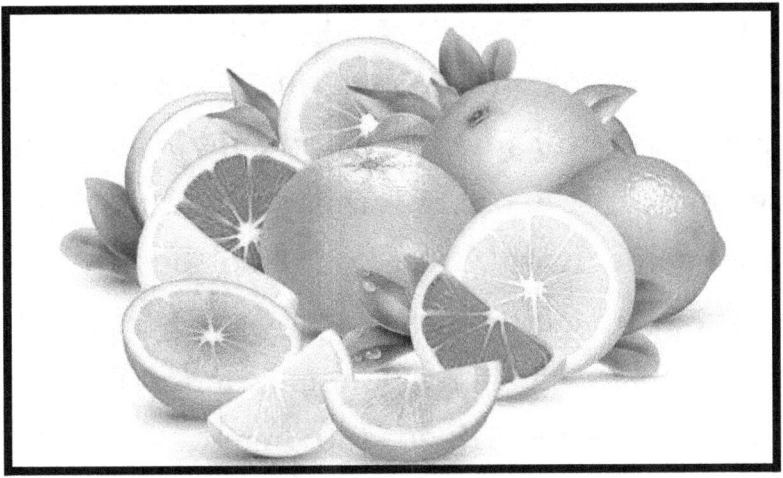

The muscle's preferred fuel during high-intensity activities such as basketball is carbohydrate. The body stores carbohydrate as glycogen in the liver and skeletal muscle. Carbohydrate stored in the liver maintains blood glucose between meals. The liver stores between 75–100 g of carbohydrate, enough to maintain blood glucose during a 12- hour fast. Most people have used up the majority of their liver glycogen by the time they awaken in the morning, which is why it's so important for athletes to eat before morning practice

Skeletal muscle stores an additional 300–400 g of carbohydrate. Unlike liver glycogen, the muscle uses its supply of carbs to fuel exercise, and training can nearly double the amount of glycogen the muscle can store. This is advantageous because the more glycogen in the muscle, the longer an athlete can sprint, jump, and run. When muscle glycogen stores are full, most athletes have enough to fuel 90–100 minutes of high-intensity activity. Terms such as "hitting the wall"

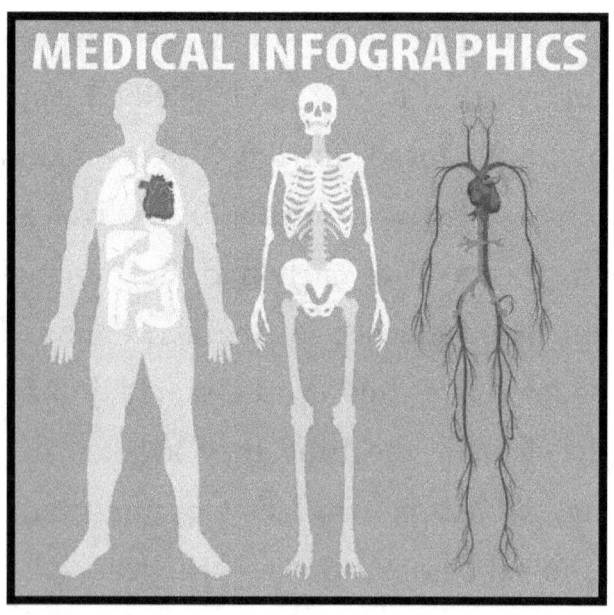

or "bonking" are used to describe the phenomenon that happens when an athlete's glycogen stores run low. While individual practices and games may not be enough to deplete muscle glycogen, inadequate carbohydrate intake coupled with daily training can deplete muscle glycogen over the course of several days. This leaves a player fatigued or with a feeling of "heavy legs."

Basketball players should consume a high-carbohydrate diet; that is to say that at least 55% of total calories in the diet should come from food rich in carbohydrate such as fruits, vegetables, bread, pasta, and rice. Most sports dietitians recommend carbohydrate intake based on body mass to ensure an athlete consumes adequate energy from carbohydrate. The range of intake suggested for basketball players is 5–7 (and up to 10) g/kg body weight (see sample diet below). The amount will vary depending upon playing time and the time of year (preseason, in-season, or postseason).

Protein

Protein is important for building and maintaining lean body mass. Although many athletes take supplements and make efforts to increase dietary protein to build muscle mass, this is usually unnecessary if they are eating a well-balanced diet with sufficient energy and protein intake spaced throughout the day. The following recipes can be used to help add protein and calories to your diet. If lactose intolerant, substitute lactose-free milk, soy milk, cashew milk, coconut milk, almond milk. Consult with your doctor before adding protein or more calories to your diet.

Peachy Cinnamon Shake
- 1 cup canned peaches
- ½ cup plain Greek yogurt
- ½ cup milk
- 1 tablespoon honey
- ½ teaspoon of cinnamon
- 3 ice cubes

276 calories, 17 g protein

Pineapple-Coconut Smoothie
- 1 cup pineapple
- ½ cup milk
- ½ cup Greek yogurt
- 1 tablespoon coconut
- 1 frozen banana, sliced

379 calories, 16 g protein

A player that weighs 82 kg (180 lb) may need up to 150 g. While eating protein above this amount is not harmful to healthy people, it often displaces energy from carbohydrates in the diet, which, as discussed above, is the muscle's preferred fuel. While the muscles will utilize protein when carbohydrate levels are low, this is an inefficient metabolic process and will leave the athlete feeling run down and fatigued. The recommendation for daily protein intake for basketball players is 1.4–1.7 g/kg of body mass.

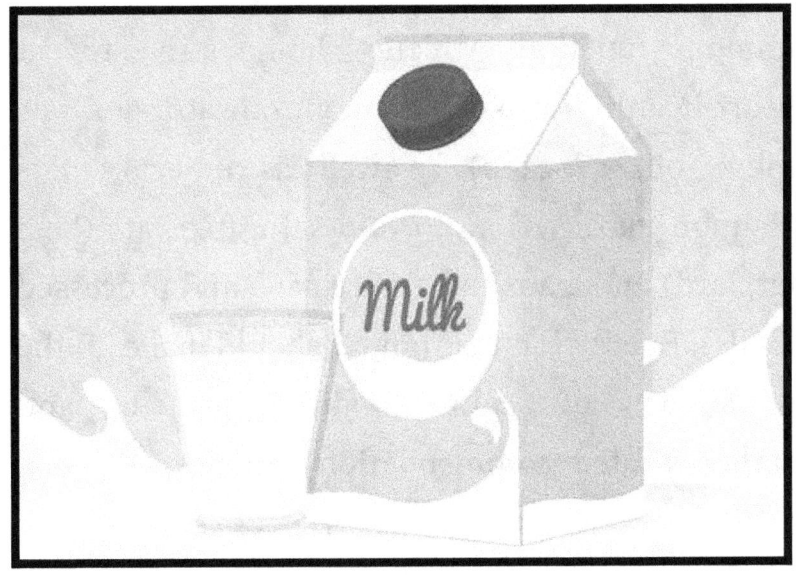

Fat

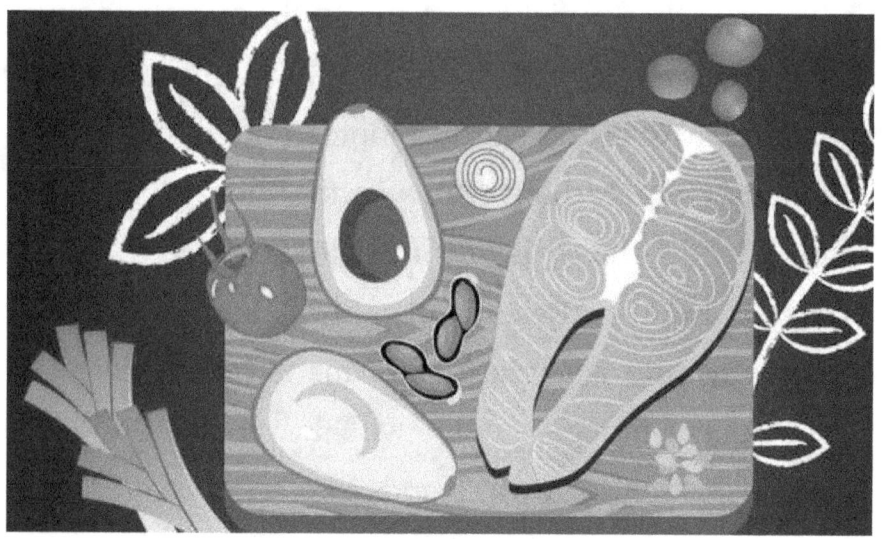

Dietary fats are important for the synthesis of hormones and cell membranes, as well as proper immune function. Athletes should strive to eat heart-healthy fats such as mono-unsaturated fats (olive oil, avocado) as well as omega-3 fats (salmon, flaxseed) and avoid saturated fats (beef fat, lard) and trans fats (margarine and processed foods). Energy intake from fat should make up the remainder of calories after protein and carbohydrate recommendations are met.

Pregame Meals

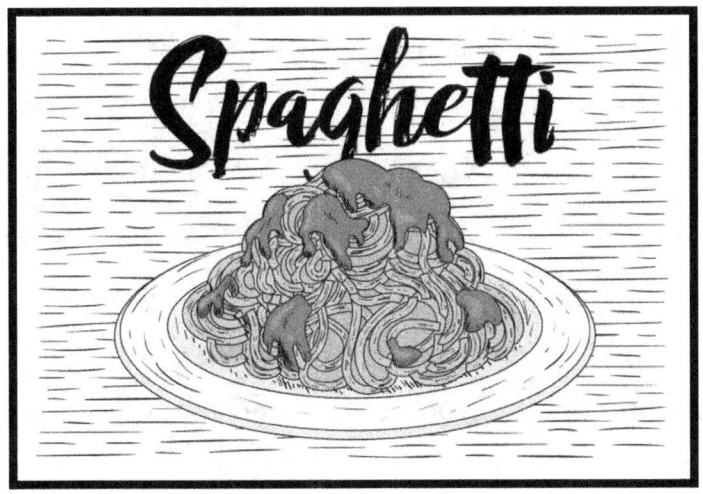

The goal for any pre-competition meal is to support the body's energy needs (e.g., top off liver glycogen) while eliminating the distraction of hunger and reducing the risk of gastrointestinal problems. Appropriate meals or foods should be high in carbohydrate, low in fat, and low in fiber. A good rule of thumb for incorporating carbohydrate is the following equation:

(bodyweight in kilograms) x (hours prior to competition) = grams of carbohydrate

For example, a player weighing 68 kg (150 lb) and eating 3 hours prior to the game could eat: 68 kg x 3 hours = 204 grams of carbohydrate This would be equivalent to a small meal including a turkey sandwich, an ounce of pretzels, a granola bar, and 1 L (33 oz) of Gatorade Thirst Quencher. On the other hand, if this player is eating 1 hour prior to the game, only about 70 g of carbohydrate should be consumed. An appropriate snack may be 1 liter (33 oz) of Gatorade Thirst Quencher and an ounce of pretzels. It is very important that each player find which foods and beverages work best for her or him by experimenting before and during practices. Each person is a bit different, and one player's "lucky" meal may leave a teammate with stomach cramps.

Fueling During Games

Basketball games last 32–48 minutes of total playing time, depending on the level. Although it is unlikely that a player will drain his muscle and liver glycogen stores, supplementing with carbohydrate during the game may help maintain performance in the fourth quarter. Research shows that both cognitive function[5] and sprint speed[1] are maintained in basketball-type protocols when subjects are supplemented with carbohydrate rather than a placebo. Again, players should experiment during practices to find what foods and beverages work best for them; however, Thirst Quencher, sports gels or chews, portions of sports bars, or oranges have been used by many. The recommended amount of carbohydrate to consume to maintain performance is 30–60 g/h. Therefore, given the game duration, an athlete should find the best solution to take in 30–60 g of carbohydrate over the course of a game. Using Gatorade Thirst Quencher, for example, 16–32 oz will meet the carbohydrate needs and provide fluid and electrolytes.

Importantly, all forms of carbohydrate supplementation should also include fluid replacement, as dehydration is detrimental to basketball performance. Fortunately, basketball lends itself to natural breaks in the action. Time-outs, breaks between quarters, and halftime are opportunities for players to refuel and rehydrate. As mentioned previously, consuming foods or fluids should be practiced during training to determine the most effective strategy. To determine an individual's sweat rate, weigh your players before and after a practice session in the same clothing, after toweling off excess sweat. If they lost weight, they didn't drink enough fluid and should consume an additional 16 oz per pound of body weight lost in the next practice. Each player should aim to lose < 2% body weight during practices and games (e.g., 3 lbs, for a 150-lb, player), and the amount that each player will need to maintain hydration will be different. Likewise, each player may prefer and tolerate different forms of carbohydrate. Players should be encouraged to find the combination of foods and fluids that works best to maintain hydration and energy while reducing the risk of stomach cramps.

Recovery

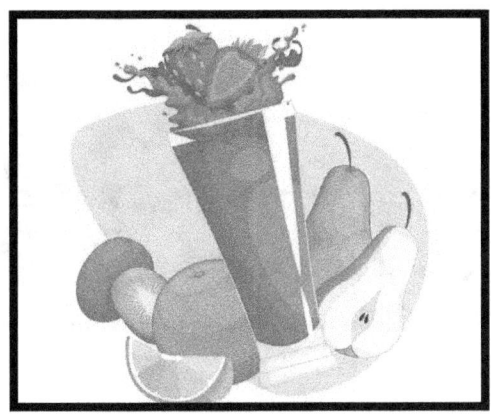

Recovery nutrition is very important when players have less than 24 hours between games or training sessions. In the 30–60 minutes immediately following exercise, the muscles used during exercise are especially sensitive to amino acids and glucose in the blood and are able to use them for muscle protein synthesis and glycogen restoration, respectively. Eating a meal or drinking a recovery shake during this "window" of time allows the muscle to recover its glycogen stores much more quickly than the same meal eaten 2 or 3 hours after exercise.

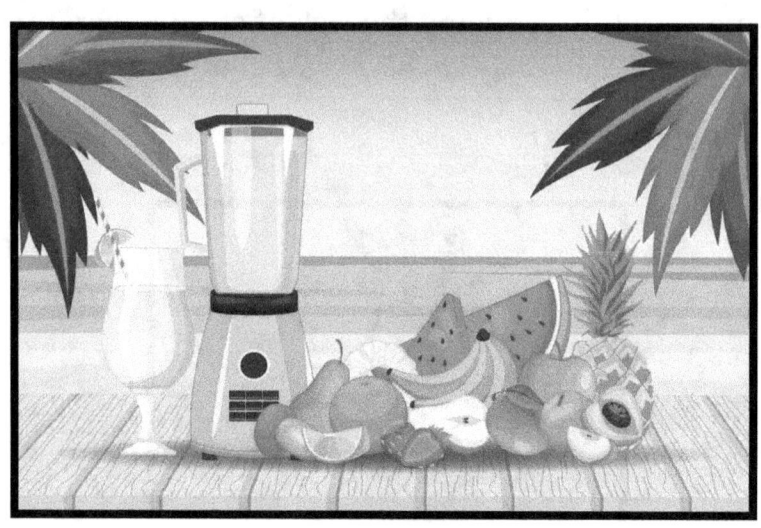

Recommended carbohydrate intake is 1.0–1.2 g of carbohydrate/kg body weight and about 20 g protein. For a 68 kg (150-lb.) person, this would be about 82 g carbohydrate (328 kcal). Some players prefer liquid meals for recovery, as they may not have an appetite following competition.

Many commercial recovery products are available; however, chocolate milk and other foods are also appropriate.

Although it is important to consume carbohydrate and protein during the time immediately following competition, players should make a point of eating a well-balanced meal within 2 hours to give the muscles another "dose" of fuel. Athletes should also rehydrate after practices and games with about 20–24 oz, of fluid, preferably with sodium, for every pound of body weight lost.

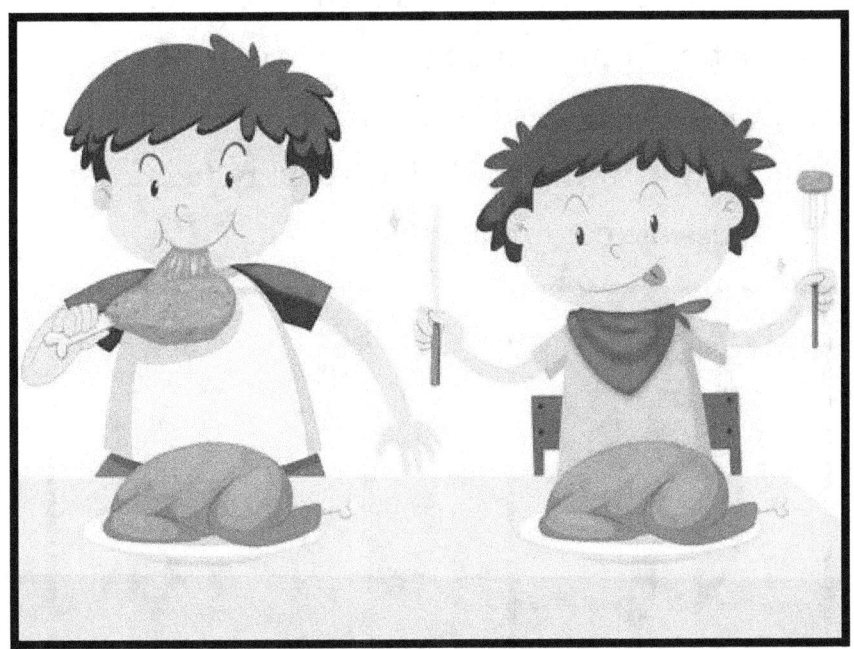

Developing the skills needed to become a great basketball player requires dedication to hours of time spent shooting, passing, ball-handling, and conditioning. Ignoring proper nutrition is like building a high- performance sports car and putting the wrong gas in the tank; it cannot operate optimally unless its engine is given high-grade fuel. Such is the case with athletes. Although the body can function on "junk food," it will not perform as well as it could when given the proper types of food; in the correct amounts; at the optimal times. Eating a variety of whole grain, fruit and vegetables, lean sources of protein, and healthy fats will provide high-quality fuel for the best possible performance.

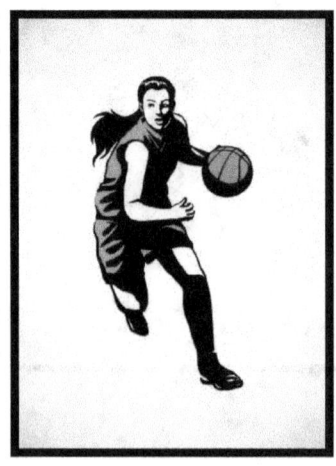 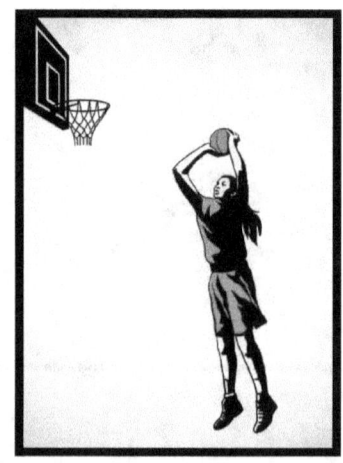

Agility Drills
(Improve Jumping Ability)

Jump rope

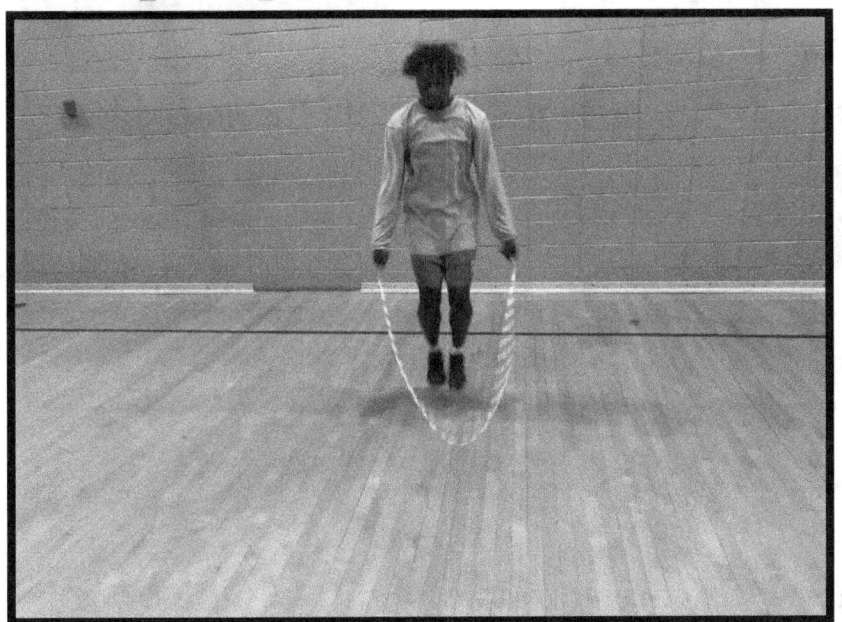

Pick the correct jump rope from any sports store.

We suggest a straightforward thick jump rope.

Get comfortable with your jump rope.

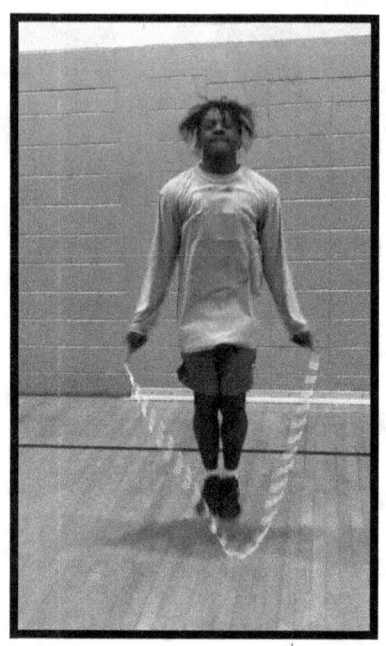 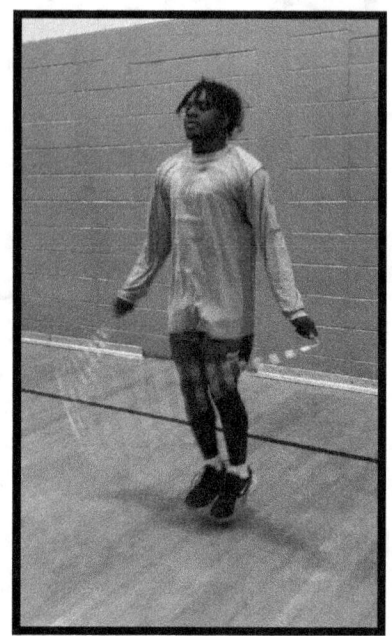

Start with your hands on both handles. Grab the handles loosely with your fingers, not your full palms.

Hold your handles with a relaxed grip.

Hold your elbows in near you body and prepare to jump.

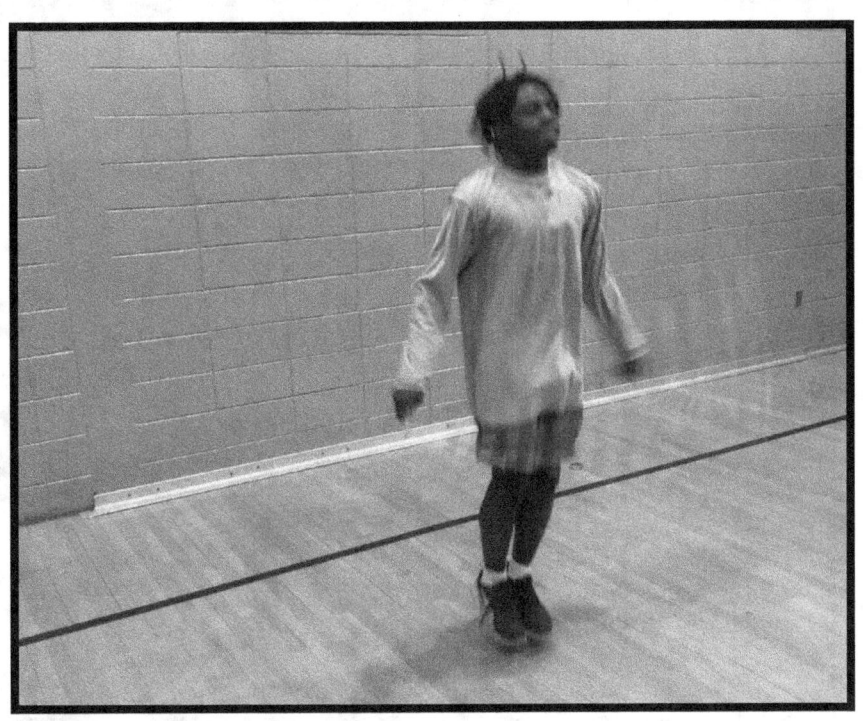

In the early stages it may look or feel funny- keep trying.

You can pretend jumping rope or try to complete a few jumps in a row.

When jumping rope you must time it almost perfect.

Jump on the top section of your feet with your back straight and your chin pointed up.

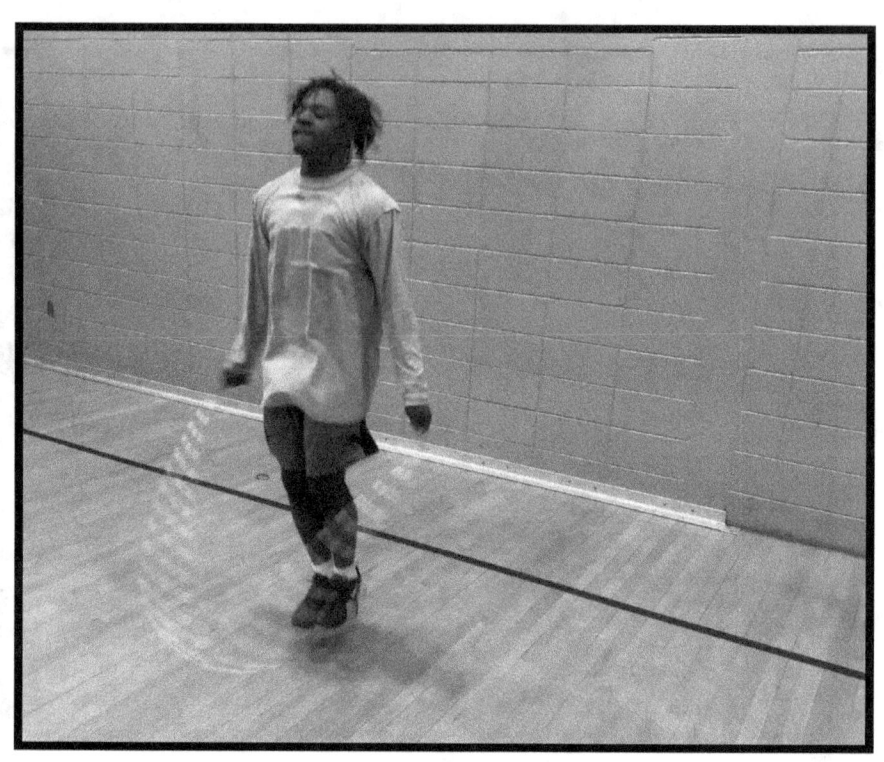

Workout Plan

Week one: Start off with ten jumps daily for seven straight days.

Week two: Pick up the pace and complete twenty-five jumps three times a week.

Week three: Fifty jumps three times a week without messing up you count.

Box Jumps

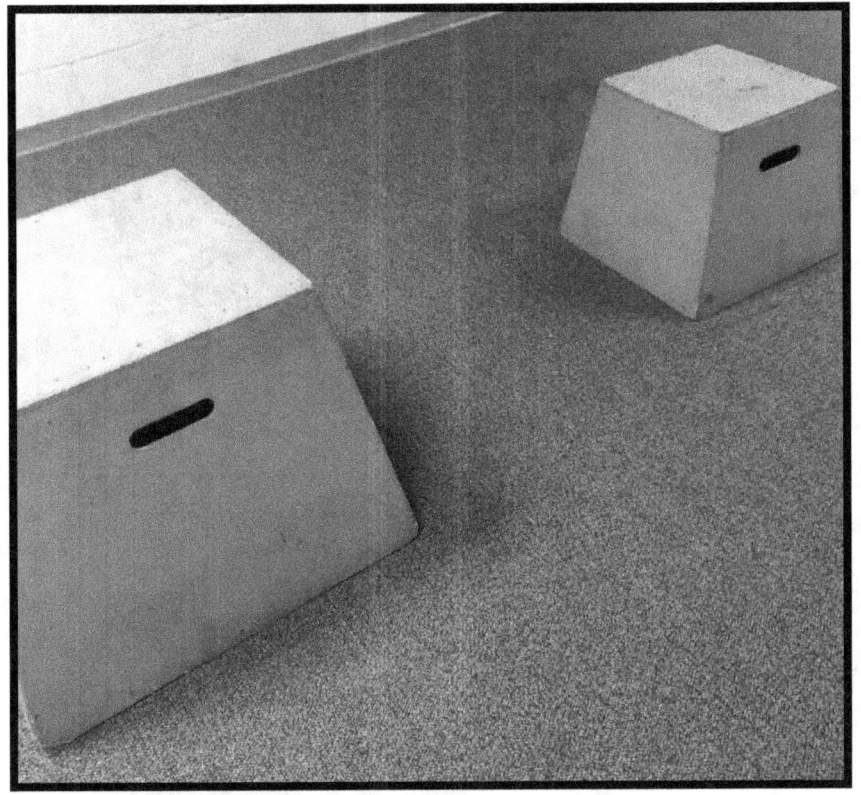

Pick the best boxes to start off slow. We suggest small boxes and working your way up.

Make sure your boxes are stable and sturdy.

Get comfortable with the boxes.

Box Jumps Workout

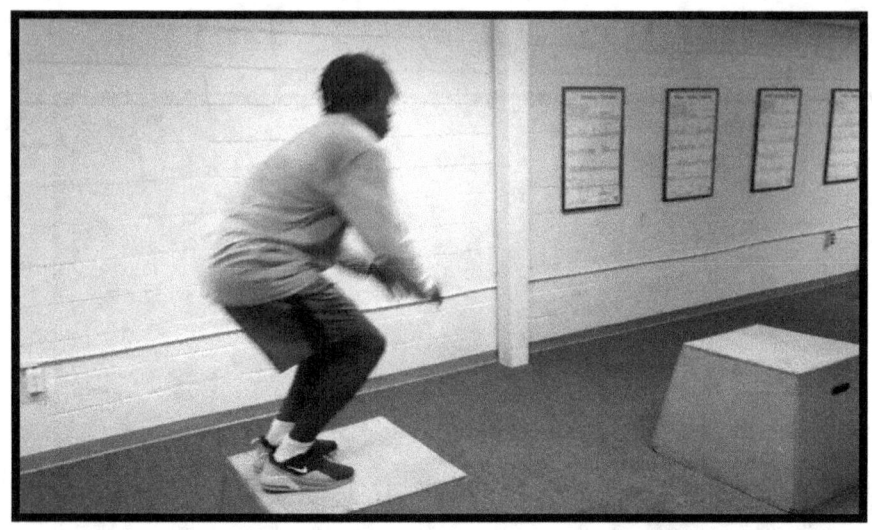

Start close to your first box, then jump up and land softly on your first box.

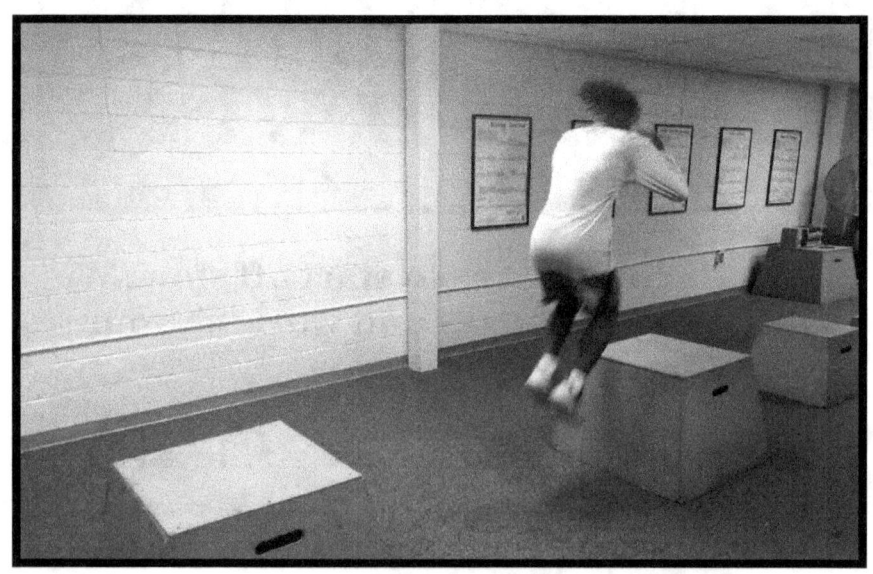

Jump down from box one to the floor. Next, jump from the floor onto the next box.

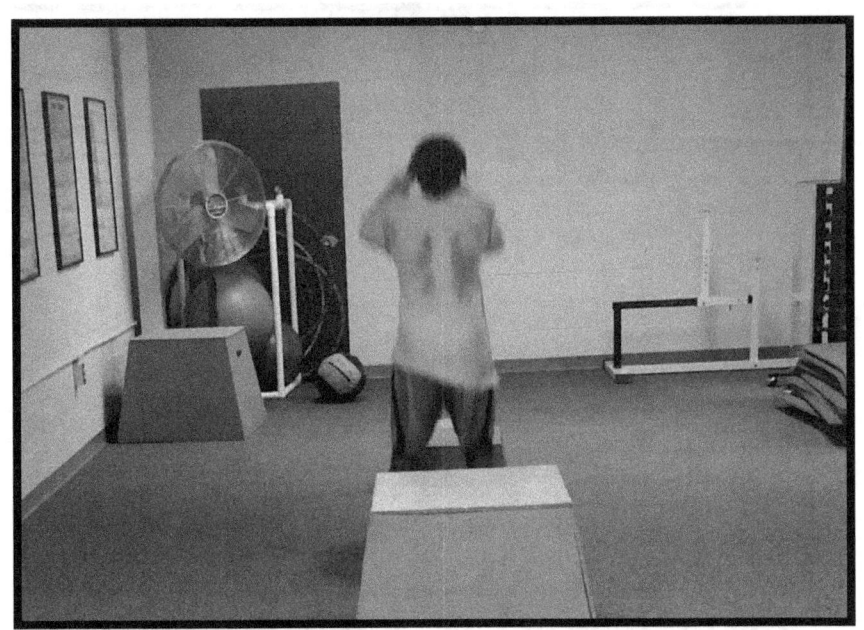

Jump down from the next box to the floor. Continue until you have completed the series of boxes.

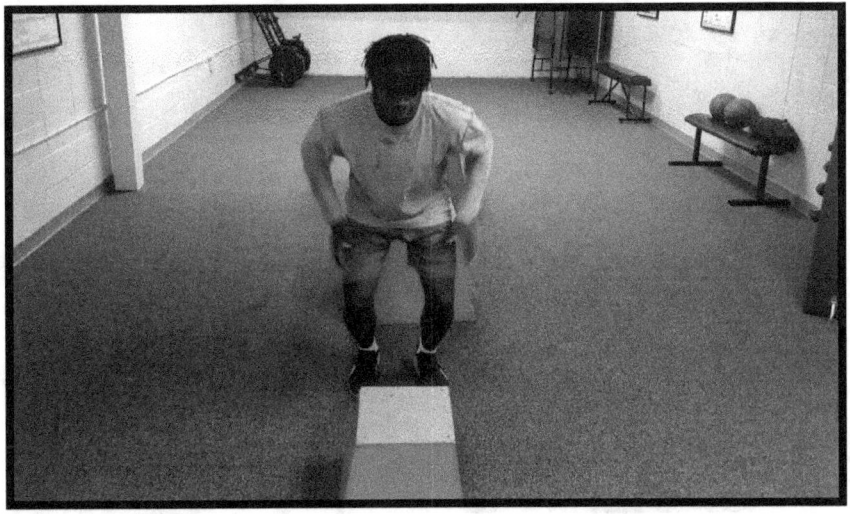

Next, turn around and start the process over in reverse.

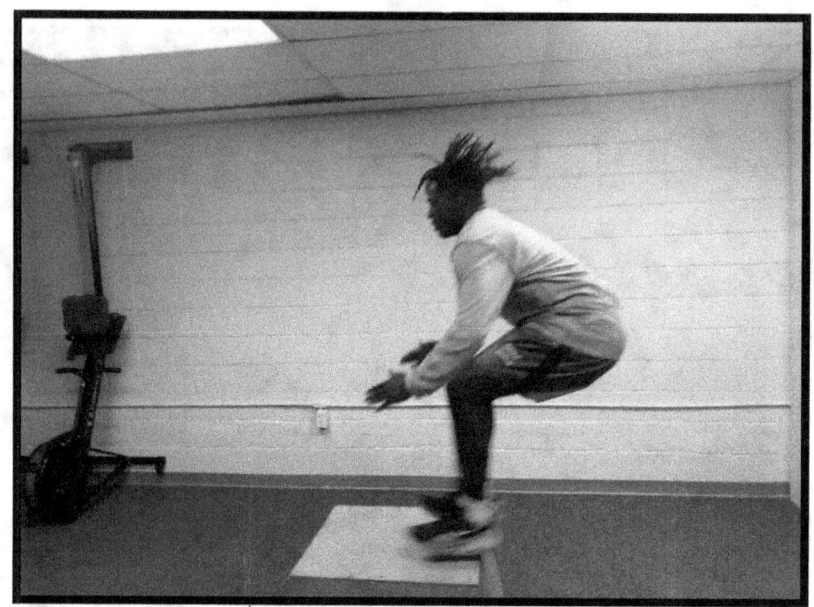

Begin close to box - jump up and land softly on your first box. Continue as with first series.

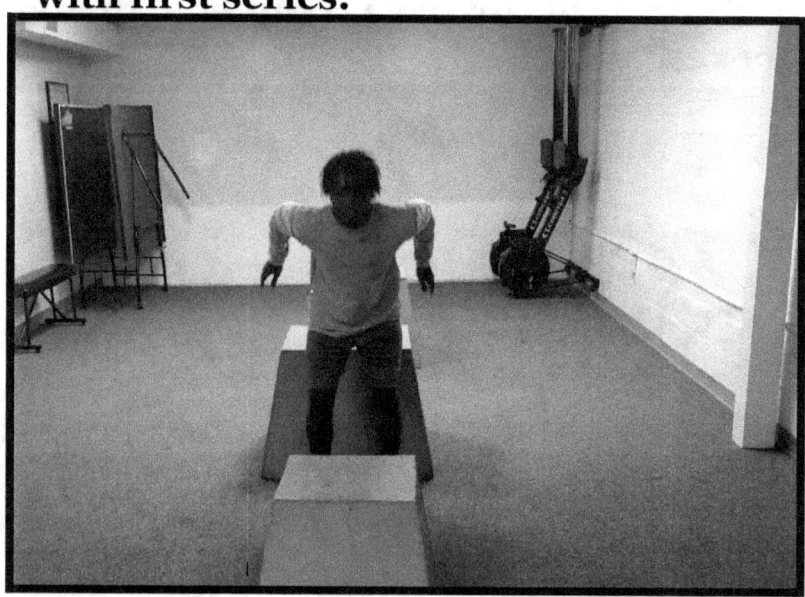

Finally, jump onto your last box then to the floor and your cycle is complete.

Conclusion

If you're looking for a physical activity to get your child off the couch, basketball is a sport that your any child can start at an early age. Playing basketball helps children learn basic coordination and team-building skills with an added bonus of making new friends along the way. Getting your child going with basic basketball skills at a young age not only helps encourage exercise, but serves as a foundation for staying active later in life.

Some basketball programs begin for children as young as 5 years old. For young children, programs focus on developing basic skills and typically use shorter 6-foot rims. Rule-based play typically does not begin until kids are 7 to 9 years old. By fourth or fifth grade, many kids are ready to play basketball against other teams. In addition to coach-supervised basketball camps, kids can practice at home to stay active.

Children ages 6 to 17 require at least one hour of moderate intensity physical activity every day.

Kids should engage in vigorous-intensive physical activity three days each week, according to the Centers for Disease Control and Prevention. Learning basketball allows children to incorporate frequent physical activity into their daily routines and contributes to overall physical well-being and fitness.

Learning to play basketball involves dribbling, throwing, catching and pivoting. Beginning basketball training at a young age improves gross motor skills by using major muscle groups. Young children who play basketball improve flexibility and endurance. Your child will also benefit from improved fine motor skills, such as hand-eye coordination. These motor skills transfer to other activities of daily life.

Becoming involved with basketball at an early age helps kids develop psychologically. Playing on a team allows your child to make friends and feel involved with her peer group. Team sports also improve a child's ability to communicate and solve basic problems. Experiencing the benefits and difficulties of healthy competition at a young age prepare children for failures later in life. Basketball teaches children social skills and coping strategies that are useful at school, home and in peer relationships.

For many people, playing basketball is a fun and effective form of exercise. While other vigorous aerobic activities offer some of the same benefits, the additional advantages basketball offers makes it an enjoyable and even important part of their lifestyles. If you've never played basketball before, consider joining a recreational team or inviting a few friends out to a public park for a quick game.

Basketball Stats

Player	#	Points	Rebounds	Assists	Steals

Notes

Blocks	Turnovers	Fouls	Total Points

Basketball Stats

Player	#	Points	Rebounds	Assists	Steals

Notes

Blocks	Turnovers	Fouls	Total Points

Basketball Stats

Player	#	Points	Rebounds	Assists	Steals

Notes

Blocks	Turnovers	Fouls	Total Points

_____

_____

_____

_____

_____

_____

_____

Basketball Stats

Player	#	Points	Rebounds	Assists	Steals

Notes

Blocks	Turnovers	Fouls	Total Points

Basketball Stats

Player	#	Points	Rebounds	Assists	Steals

Notes

Blocks	Turnovers	Fouls	Total Points

Basketball Stats

Player	#	Points	Rebounds	Assists	Steals

Notes

Blocks	Turnovers	Fouls	Total Points

Basketball Stats

Player	#	Points	Rebounds	Assists	Steals

Notes

Blocks	Turnovers	Fouls	Total Points

Basketball Stats

Player	#	Points	Rebounds	Assists	Steals

Notes

Blocks	Turnovers	Fouls	Total Points

Basketball Stats

Player	#	Points	Rebounds	Assists	Steals

Notes

Blocks	Turnovers	Fouls	Total Points

Basketball Stats

Player	#	Points	Rebounds	Assists	Steals

Notes

Blocks	Turnovers	Fouls	Total Points

Disclaimer Statement

All information and content contained in this book are provided solely for general information and reference purposes. SSP LLC Limited makes no statement, representation, warranty or guarantee as to the accuracy, reliability or timeliness of the information and content contained in this Book.

Neither SSP Limited or the author of this book nor any of its related company accepts any responsibility or liability for any direct or indirect loss or damage (whether in tort, contract or otherwise) which may be suffered or occasioned by any person howsoever arising due to any inaccuracy, omission, misrepresentation or error in respect of any information and content provided by this book (including any third-party books. Consult with your doctor before staring any drill or workout connected to this book.

www.ingramcontent.com/pod-product-compliance
Lightning Source LLC
Chambersburg PA
CBHW072020110526
44592CB00012B/1380